Homeopathy

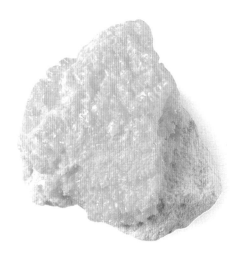

Homeopathy

A Beginner's Guide to Natural Remedies for Use in the Home

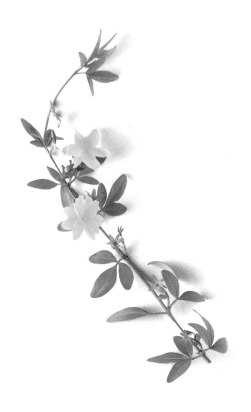

Sylvia Treacher

SMITHMARK

Distributed in the USA by SMITHMARK Publishers,
a division of U.S. Media Holdings Inc.,
16, East 32nd Street, New York, NY 10016

First published in the UK in 1996

SMITHMARK books are available for bulk purchase for sales promotion and premium use. For details, write or call the
manager of special sales, SMITHMARK Publishers, 16 East 32nd Street, New York NY 10016; (212) 532-6600

ISBN: 0-7651-9814-2

1 0 9 8 7 6 5 4 3 2 1

Edited, designed and produced by Haldane Mason

Editor: Maggi McCormick
Special Photography: Amanda Heywood
Illustrator: Jack McCarthy

Colour reproduction by Regent Publishing Services, Hong Kong

Picture Acknowledgements
Mary Evans Picture Library: 7, 8, 9 (top); **NHPA:** © Daniel Heuclin 60; **Oxford Scientific Films:** © Deni Brown 68,
© Michael Fogden 71, © David G. Fox 57, © Zig Leszczynski 65, © James Robinson 55.

The author and publishers would like to thank Helios Pharmacy in Ashford, Kent, for their help in the preparation of
this book.

IMPORTANT

The information, recipes and remedies contained in this book are generally applicable and appropriate in most
cases, but are not tailored to specific circumstances or individuals. Any of the substances can produce an allergic
reaction, and the author and publishers cannot be held responsible for any problems arising from the mistaken
identity of any plants or remedies, or the inappropriate use of any remedy or healing regime. Homeopathic
remedies should be taken as part of a complete system of medicine under the guidance of a qualified homeopathic
practitioner. Do not undertake any form of self diagnosis or treatment for serious complaints without first seeking
professional advice. Always seek professional medical advice if symptoms persist.

NOTE

Certain spellings used in this book may not be familiar to all readers, so here is a list of common alternatives:

anaemia = anemia	anaesthetic = anesthetic	Caesarean = Cesarean
diarrhoea = diarrhea	foetus = fetus	gonorrhoea = gonorrhea
gynaecological = gynecological	haemoglobin = hemoglobin	haemorrhage = hemorrhage
haemorrhoids = hemorrhoids	leucorrhoea = leucorrhea	oedematous = edematous
oesophagus = esophagus	pharmacopoeia = pharmacopeia	

Contents

What is Homeopathy?

HOMEOPATHY IS A SYSTEM OF MEDICINE which powerfully stimulates the body's own healing mechanism to reinstate health and well-being. Around the body is an electro-magnetic energy field, or aura, which can be seen by some people, and this is where homeopathic medicines have their primary action. This energy animates all life and departs at death. It is called *chi* in Chinese Medicine and in Sanskrit, *prana*, which means breath or vital force. All matter consists of atoms which vibrate at different speeds. Homeopathy is the art and skill of matching the vibration, or energy, of the remedy to that of the person. Symptoms of illness are a vibrational language, therefore, which help the homeopath to select the most curative medicines.

Over the last ten to fifteen years there has been a strong movement towards the idea of taking responsibility for our own health, which has resulted in a huge demand for methods of healing which take a look at the whole person – emotionally and mentally, as well as physically. There has been a subsequent growth in the popularity of homeopathy which has resulted in a much wider availability of remedies in health-food shops, pharmacies and supermarkets.

It can be used very effectively in self-prescribing for treating accidents and minor ailments as long as the basic principles are adhered to. These are described on the following pages. Because many homeopathic remedies have a vast range of applications, it may be confusing to go into a shop and find some containers labelled for specific ailments, such as headache or indigestion; for example, Carbo Veg can be given to alleviate flatulent bloating, but it can also be used in an emergency situation where there is collapse and difficulty in breathing. For best results, remedies need to be matched to a group of symptoms, as short-cut methods may lead to disappointment. But in some first aid situations, remedies will work when chosen on one leading symptom only, such as Arnica for bruising.

Homeopathic remedies are usually sold in tablet form but can also be bought as powders and tinctures. Tablets are easy to administer and are dissolved under the tongue. Although there are no conventional side effects, accidental 'provings' are possible. If homeopathic remedies are taken unwisely and repeated when no longer required, the symptoms for which the remedy was originally taken may return.

This book describes how to apply homeopathic medicines to relieve pain, swelling, shock, promote the fast healing of wounds and sprains, and even soothe teething babies. Ordeals such as examinations, dental treatment and surgery are included, as well as jet travel, with suggestions to help you recover from jetlag, sunstroke, frostbite or insect stings. Remedies to help some mental and emotional upsets are also given. Long-term illness is not dealt with here, because these require regular visits to a homeopath for constitutional prescribing, but the acute stages of some chronic complaints are.

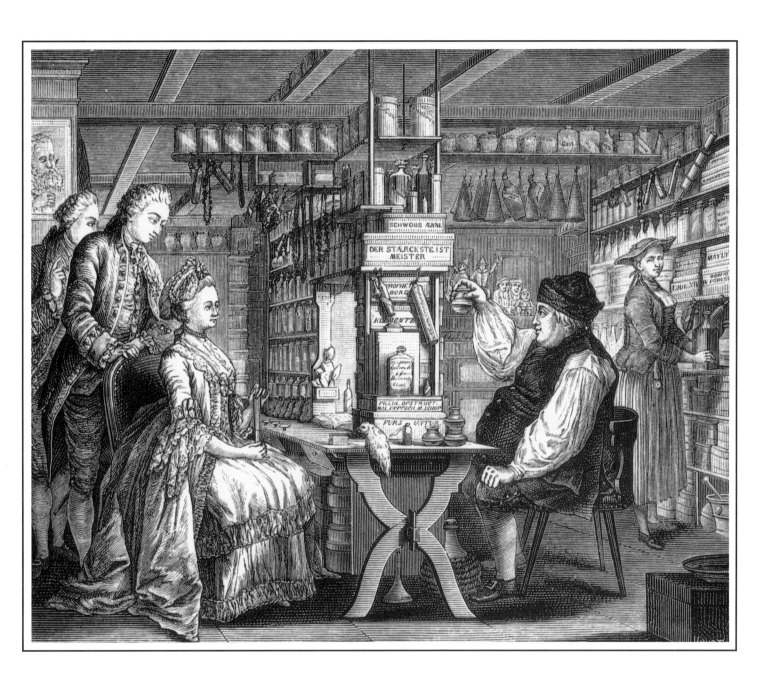

Receiving treatment at a Swiss rural pharmacy in 1774.
Homeopaths draw up a personal profile of their patients,
including family medical history, to treat the body as a
whole. When prescribing remedies, a homeopath takes into
account all aspects of a person's life, as an illness may be the
result of a wide variety of causes, both physical or mental.

Principles and Background

The foundations of this healing system rest very firmly on principles which can be summed up as follows: Like Cures Like (The Law of Similars); Totality of Symptoms; Minimum Dose; Single Remedy; Direction of Cure.

Remedies

The medicines are referred to as remedies and are made from substances obtained mostly from plants and minerals, and some from the animal kingdom, including some poisons. They are normally taken in the form of small white pills which are dissolved under the tongue and they can also be obtained as tinctures or powders. The knowledge of how to use the remedies comes from three main sources: 'provings', poisonings and clinical experience.

Samuel Hahnemann (1755–1843).

Provings

This is the term used when a substance is tested on healthy adult volunteers. (Remedies are never tested on animals.) The remedy being proved is normally given in repeated doses to a group of people until symptoms occur; a detailed record is kept of each person's experience and this information is eventually incorporated into the homeopathic materia medicas.

Totality of symptoms and finding the appropriate remedy

To find the appropriate remedy, the overall symptom picture must be taken into account before the most similar remedy is chosen to match the person's complaint; this is called finding the similimum. It is not necessary to match all the symptoms of a remedy. For the purposes of first aid, the physical symptoms of the person need to be matched as closely as possible to information on the physical symptoms of the remedy. However, if the remedy itself has a strong 'personality' picture, this should also be taken into account.

The law of similars

In the 4th century BC, the Greek physician Hippocrates found that there were two distinct approaches to illness – one way by 'opposites' and the other by 'similars'. Orthodox medicine – or allopathy – heals by 'opposites', and homeopathy heals by 'similars'. The words 'allopathy' and 'homeopathy' are both from the Greek and mean 'opposite suffering' and 'similar suffering' respectively.

For example, orthodox medicine gives analgesics to 'kill' the pain of a headache, which act by inhibiting the nerve sensations. By contrast, in homeopathy a remedy is chosen which has that pain as part of its symptom picture; if repeatedly given to a healthy person, or someone not suffering that pain, eventually they would develop it. A child poisoned by eating berries of the Belladonna plant would develop a high fever with dry burning heat, possibly hallucinate and have dilated pupils with light sensitivity. In a sick person with these symptoms, one of the first homeopathic remedies to be considered is Belladonna.

It was the German physician and chemist Samuel Hahnemann (1755–1843) who brilliantly drew together the principles of homeopathy. Hahnemann had become disillusioned with the medical practices of his day and while translating a medical text on the treatment of malaria, he disagreed with the author and decided to experiment on himself. By taking crude doses of Peruvian Bark (Cinchona Bark from which quinine is derived), he brought out symptoms similar to those of malaria, which disappeared as soon as he discontinued taking it. In this way he established the first principle, Like Cures Like or The Law of Similars.

Minimum dose

Because of Hahnemann's great efforts to reduce the poisonous effects of large doses of medicines in use at that time, such as mercury in the treatment of syphillis, he investigated diluting them. During this time, he discovered that if the medicines were mixed vigorously by striking the bottle against a firm surface (succussion), they became stronger in their effects, even though there was less of the original substance because of dilution. After several years his diligence eventually led to the establishment

A 15th-century German pharmaceutical lesson.

of another major principle of homeopathy, that of the Minimum Dose.

Single dose

Homeopaths normally give one remedy at a time. This tradition dates back to the sound principles which Hahnemann laid down. His experience showed that it was impossible to assess the outcome accurately if several medicines were given simultaneously. Much information in the homeopathic materia medicas comes from data gathered over the last 150–200 years, mainly from provings of single substances and chemical compounds, and is as applicable now as it was then.

Direction of cure

Constantine Hering, a pupil of Hahnemann, noticed that symptoms of illness moved in a particular direction as cure was being achieved. He observed that disease moved from the inside to the outside, from very important organs to less important organs (e.g. if an asthmatic child who previously had eczema was treated homeopathically, the asthma would improve as the eczema returned), and in the reverse order in which they appeared. This is known as the Direction of Cure and is the last of the four principles.

To summarize the principles: Like Cures Like based on the Totality of Symptoms; Minimum Dose; Single Remedy; Direction of Cure.

WHY CHOOSE HOMEOPATHY?

Homeopathy is relatively straightforward to use for everyday ailments and accidents, and positive results will be obtained if a few basic rules are followed. Remedies can be given safely to newborn babies and children, and in pregnancy – with a few exceptions detailed on page 13. First aid kits can be purchased which are small and easy to keep in hand luggage when travelling, but ideally should not be put through X-ray security machines at airports.

Information is given for treating very serious accidents, as well as minor ones, because it is well known among homeopaths that remedies can reduce haemorrhage and shock in some life-threatening situations. Naturally, calling for an ambulance is still a very necessary procedure.

In acute illness, symptoms may come on suddenly or over a

few days, and they may disappear on their own without intervention of any kind, but the severity of the illness and confidence in using the remedies will determine what action is needed.

Symptoms represent the body's attempt to heal itself and are a way of saying that something is out of balance; they are an expression of lack of ease (dis-ease). If health is to be restored, symptoms need to be welcomed rather than ignored or suppressed in some way. Because of its strengthening effect on the immune system, users of homeopathy find that they become less susceptible to illness in general, and to common ailments such as coughs and colds in particular, but this does require long-term prescribing from a professional. A homeopath would take into account possible causes on all levels – mental and emotional as well as physical, including habitual thought patterns, as these can create illness in the physical body; also a detailed

family medical history would be taken as a means of highlighting genetically inherited weaknesses. In the context of first aid, this would apply to someone who constantly had accidents.

While Western orthodox medicine becomes more and more complex with ever-increasing technology, homeopathy stands firm on its original foundations. People change, the environment changes – hence a continually evolving expression of disease. To find the right remedy becomes, in one sense, more complicated, because now we have several additional layers to work through which didn't exist 200 years ago – powerful drugs including antibiotics, the Pill, hormone replacement therapy, immunization, environmental pollutants, etc. For these reasons new remedies are from time to time added to the homeopathic stock.

Making Remedies

The first step in making a remedy is to produce a tincture. This is done by soaking the chosen substance in pure alcohol. Most plants yield readily to this process, as they are soluble in alcohol. Specimens are collected at particular seasons and specific parts of each plant are used according to methods of preparation recorded in standard pharmacopoeias. Some plants, as well as minerals and substances from the animal kingdom, are not readily soluble in alcohol and have to be prepared first by grinding (triturating) with lactose (milk sugar) in a pestle and mortar for several hours. After this, they become soluble and a tincture can be prepared in the same way as for alcohol-soluble plants.

The next step is to take one drop of the tincture and add it to 9 drops of alcohol. It is then shaken (succussed) a specific number of times; this produces the first dilution or potency of 1×. The × stands for the decimal scale (1 + 9 = 10). To get the next potency, one drop is taken from the 1× dilution and added to a further 9 drops of alcohol and shaken; this gives the 2× potency. If this method is continued another four times, it results in the 6× potency.

If instead of 9 drops, 99 drops of alcohol are used, this is referred to as the centesimal scale. These are the two most frequently used methods of making remedies.

TIPS FOR TAKING AND HANDLING HOMEOPATHIC REMEDIES

* Dissolve under the tongue.
* Do not swallow with a drink.
* Do not eat, drink, smoke or clean teeth for about 15 minutes before or after taking a remedy (except in urgent situations).
* Remedies should be touched as little as possible, as heat from your hand can spoil them.
* Do not transfer remedies from one container to another.
* Always throw away empty containers – do not recycle, because some of the remedy will adhere to the container.
* Keep away from all strong-smelling products such as perfume, soap, incense, mothballs, aromatherapy oils, peppermints, coffee, and anything containing menthol or eucalyptus.
* Keep away from sources of heat and light.

MAKING A 6× POTENCY
Producing a 6× potency is a simple procedure, but requires accuracy. First, one drop of the mother tincture is added to a test tube containing 9 drops of alcohol. The mixture is shaken by knocking it against the palm of the hand to give the first dilution. Next, one drop from the first test tube is added to the second tube, which also has 9 drops of alcohol in it. This is repeated for all six test tubes, resulting in the 6× potency. Finally, a few drops are added to a bottle of lactose carrier pills.

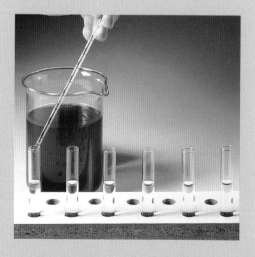

1 *Making the 1× potency or first dilution from the mother tincture.*

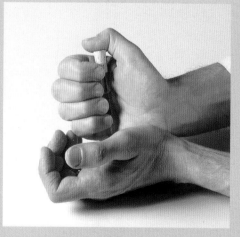

2 *Succussing (vigorously shaking) the liquid to mix the remedy thoroughly.*

If a woman takes a remedy while she is breastfeeding, her baby will receive the remedy, too. This will not do any harm and may be of benefit to the baby.

The system of halving the dose for children used in orthodox medicine does not apply to homeopathy. This is because the dilution process means that the remedies are already weak enough that they will not harm babies and young children, who can be given the same dose as an adult.

When children are too young to take pills and are likely to choke on them, crush the pills between two spoons and drop the powder into the child's mouth. Carefully sterilize spoons afterwards to avoid passing on the remedy. Alternatively, you may prefer to have a few remedies in liquid potencies (obtainable from homeopathic pharmacies). Remedies can also be given in this way to an adult where it would normally be considered dangerous to put anything solid in their mouth, for example, where the person is unconscious after fainting or collapse.

Do not panic if you find that your child has a remedy bottle open and has swallowed several pills. Normally there will be no

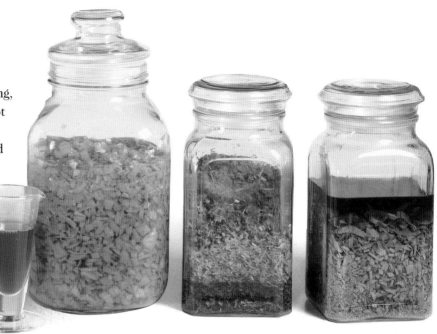

Plants are soaked in alcohol to make tinctures.

reaction because in order for homeopathy to work, remedies have to be matched to symptom pictures.

Homeopathy can be used to help older people in a variety of ways, whether to regain confidence after a fall, or to counter fear or confusion at a change in surroundings or impending surgery. Even simple irritation at their declining abilities can be alleviated by taking homeopathic remedies.

Remember: If you are already seeing a homeopath, do not take remedies without consulting your regular practitioner, unless it is an emergency, because you could interfere with your course of treatment.

Homeopathy is a system of medicine that treats the overall constitution. There are deep-acting remedies that improve people's level of susceptibility to illness, as well as remedies for acute illness and accidents. So homeopathy can help with everyday well-being as well as treating a wide range of disorders.

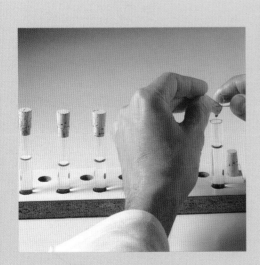

3 *One drop of the succussed remedy is placed in the next test tube for the second (2×) dilution, and so on.*

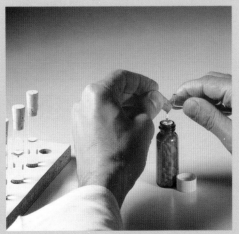

4 *The diluted, succussed remedy is added to a bottle of lactose (milk sugar) carrier pills.*

Dosage

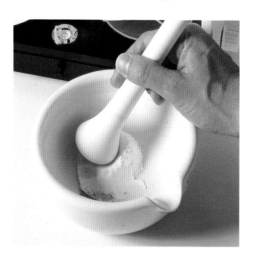

The trituration process used for some plants, minerals and animal substances involves grinding up the substance with lactose before it is made into a tincture.

There are no absolutes on how often to take the remedies and the following table is therefore for use as a general guide. Basically, the more acute or painful a situation is, the more frequently remedies can be repeated; observe the response – watch the patient, not the clock!

Giving the wrong remedy

Normally, if you give the wrong remedy, nothing happens. For homeopathy to work, your symptoms have to be matched to the symptom picture of the remedy.

If you don't get a positive result:

1 Have you chosen the right remedy?
2 Have you taken it as indicated – did you take it for long enough or change it too quickly?
3 Have you antidoted it with coffee or peppermints (see antidotes below)?

Repeating remedies

If you continue taking a remedy after your symptoms have improved, it is possible to bring your symptoms back. This will be an involuntary 'proving'. Stop taking the remedy and symptoms will usually abate. If they persist, try to antidote by drinking black coffee.

ANTIDOTES

Avoid anything with coffee, peppermint, menthol, eucalyptus and camphor, and some essential oils. (Check your toothpaste, mouthwash, etc, which may contain some antidotes.)

POTENCY TABLE

	Minor ailments	Acute	Very serious	Childbirth
	e.g. indigestion, lack of appetite, tension.	*e.g. colds, coughs, flu, fevers, earache, headache, period pains.*	*e.g. severe pain from accidents, burns, haemorrhage.*	*NB During labour, symptoms may change rapidly so several different remedies may be needed in quick succession.*
6x or 6	One twice daily for 7–10 days. Can be repeated after 2 weeks if necessary.	One every 2–4 hours for 2 days. Reduce to 3 times daily for a further 3–5 days.	One every 5–15 minutes for 6–8 doses or until relief is obtained.	One every 15–30 minutes for 3–4 doses.
30		One every 4 hours for 3 doses **only**.	One every 15–30 minutes for 4–6 doses or until relief is obtained.	One every ½–1 hour for 3–4 doses.
200			One dose only. Repeat once more **only** if clearly indicated.	One dose only – unless you are very clear it needs repeating.

There is disagreement among homeopaths about whether coffee or peppermint toothpaste really does stop remedies from working. Sometimes one cup of coffee can antidote treatment, in others it appears not to make any difference. Because remedies help healing to take place on levels which involve unseen subtle energy, we often cannot be sure if there has been an antidotal action unless the original symptoms return after having improved.

Dental treatment may also antidote the effects of remedies.

CONTRA-INDICATIONS

Do not use some remedies in the following situations:

● **Pregnancy:** Do not take Cocculus or Thuja throughout pregnancy, or Pulsatilla in the first three months.
● **After surgery or implants:** Silica (this can open up wounds).
● **History of tuberculosis:** Do not use Phosphorus, Silica or Sulphur.

REMEDIES WHICH ARE INCOMPATIBLE

The following remedies may react adversely to each other; avoid giving them in close proximity.

AFTER GIVING	DO NOT IMMEDIATELY GIVE
Calc Carb	Bryonia, Sulphur
Cantharis	Coffea
Caulophyllum	Coffea
Causticum	Cocculus, Coffea, Phosphorus
Chamomilla	Nux Vomica
Coffea	Arg Nit, Causticum, Cocculus, Ignatia
Dulcamara	Belladonna, Lachesis
Ignatia	Coffea, Tabacum
Kreosote	Carbo Veg, China
Lachesis	Dulcamara
Ledum	China
Lycopodium	Coffea
Merc Sol	Silica
Nux Vomica	Causticum, Tabacum
Nit Ac	Lachesis, Natrum Mur
Phosphorus	Apis, Causticum
Rhus Tox	Apis
Sepia	Bryonia, Lachesis
Silica	Merc Sol

FIRST AID KITS AND BIRTHING KITS

You can either select your own remedies to go into 12, 18 or 36-bottle remedy cases, or buy a ready-made kit from a homeopathic pharmacy.

Suggestions for a 12-bottle kit:

Aconite 30	Apis 30	Arnica 30
Arsenicum Album 30	Belladonna 30	Chamomilla 30
Gelsemium 30	Hypericum 30	Ledum 30
Nux Vomica 30	Pulsatilla 30	Rescue Remedy

Suggestions for an 18-bottle kit: all the above plus

Arnica 200	Baptisia 30	Bryonia 30
Hepar Sulph 30	Rhus Tox 30	Sulphur 30

Suggestions for a birthing kit:

Aconite 200	Arnica 200	Bellis Perennis 30
Calendula 30	Carbo Veg 200	Caulophyllum 200
Chamomilla 200	Cimicifuga 200	Gelsemium 200
Hypericum 200	Ipecac 200	Kali Carb 200
Kali Phos 30	Natrum Mur 200	Phosphorus 200
Pulsatilla 200	Secale 200	Staphysagria 200

Note: Reference is made in this book to Rescue Remedy and Biochemic Tissue Salts.

● Rescue Remedy is one of the 38 Bach Flower Remedies on sale in health-food shops. This is a method of healing devised by Dr Edward Bach, a physician and bacteriologist.

● The Biochemic Tissue Salts were considered by a German homeopath, Dr Schuessler, to be vitally necessary for the healthy functioning of cell activity in the body; they are used widely by some homeopaths. They are also on sale in many health-food shops.

The salts are: Calc Fluor, Calc Phos, Calc Sulph, Ferr Phos, Kali Mur, Kali Phos, Kali Sulph, Mag Phos, Nat Mur, Nat Phos, Nat Sulph, Silica.

Home-made Calendula Mother Tincture

INGREDIENTS

50 g/2 oz fresh marigolds or
25 g/1 oz dried
100 ml/3½ fl oz alcohol (use
brandy or vodka – surgical spirit,
industrial spirit and rubbing
alcohol are not suitable)

UTENSILS

pestle & mortar
chopping board
sharp knife
electric blender (optional)
fine sieve (strainer)
paper filters or muslin (cheesecloth)
small funnel
large earthenware bowl or glass container
1 large airtight glass container
(preferably dark glass)
20 ml/¾ fl oz dark glass bottles
(obtainable from pharmacists)
labels
pressure cooker (optional)

If special care is taken to sterilize utensils first, the life of the tincture will be extended. You can sterilize utensils using one of the following methods:

❋ Bring to the boil in water and simmer for 15 minutes, or

❋ Place utensils in a cool oven (110°C/225°F/Gas Mark ¼) for 40 minutes, or

❋ Place in a pressure cooker for 15 minutes, or

❋ Place in nursery sterilizing fluid.

Calendula mother tincture is ideal for home use – it can be used to bathe cuts and wounds, as a mouthwash, or to halt a haemorrhage in the mouth, for example after dental work, as well as to sooth a burnt tongue.

There are two methods that can be used to make a mother tincture at home. The best method, shown in the step pictures opposite, is more time-consuming, but worth the extra effort as it lasts for longer. A quicker method is given below.

The flowers you need to make this tincture are *Calendula officinalis* (pot marigold). To make Hypericum Mother Tincture, follow any of these methods using *Hypericum perfoliatum* (St John's Wort). For Calendula mother tincture, only the flowers, either fresh or dried, are used; for Hypericum mother tincture, use both the leaves and flowers of the fresh plant.

QUICK METHOD

This tincture will have a shorter shelf life than that made by the method showin opposite, but is simple and quick to do.

1 Make an infusion by adding 600ml/1 pint/2½ cups boiling water to the marigold flowers in a saucepan (do not use an aluminium one). Cover and leave to stand until it has cooled.

2 Strain when cool, first through a fine sieve (strainer), then through a paper filter or through muslin (cheesecloth).

3 Add 1 teaspoon of brandy or vodka to each 20 ml/¾ fl oz bottle.

4 Pour the infusion into the bottles, filling each to the top to exclude air.

HOW TO MAKE CALENDULA MOTHER TINCTURE

1 Measure out the ingredients. Wash the flowers, then pulverize them by chopping finely and grinding in the pestle and mortar. Add the flowers to the bowl and mix thoroughly with the alcohol. A quicker method is to put the flowers and alcohol into an electric blender for 1–2 minutes.

2 Pour the mixture into a large, airtight container such as a large glass jar. Fill it completely so that air is excluded and store in a cool, dark place, until the liquid turns a dark brown. If the container is clear glass, care must be taken to keep it completely dark.

3 Agitate the container regularly every day for 1 week; the liquid at the base of the jar will darken – this is the tincture.

4 After 1 week, strain through a fine sieve. Strain a second time through muslin or a paper filter. Fill small glass bottles to the top to exclude air. Label and date. Store the bottles in a cool dark place (but **not** the refrigerator).

1

2

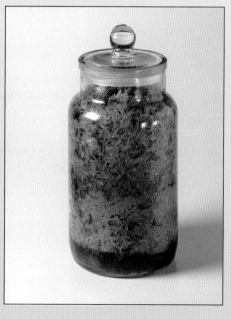

3

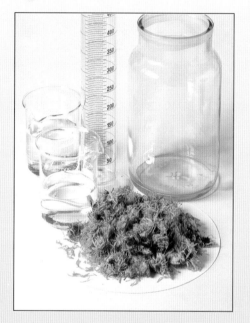

4

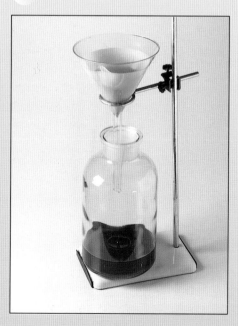

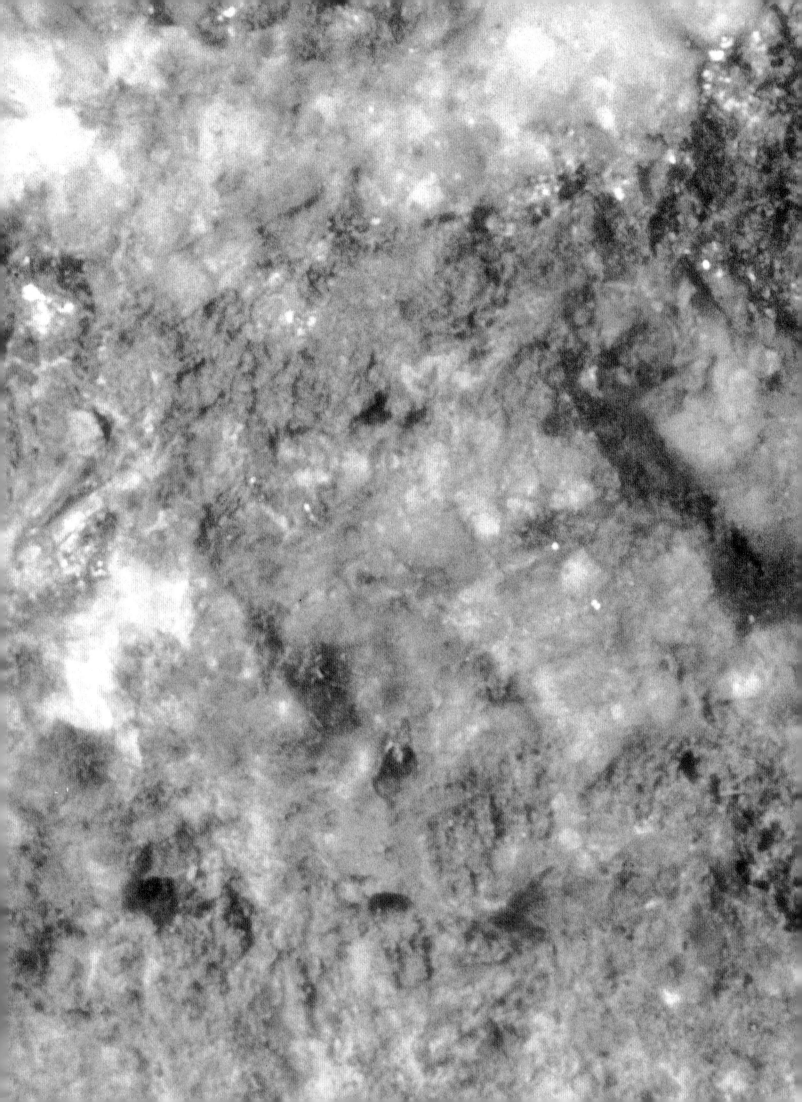

A–Z OF FIRST AID
& AILMENTS

This section gives an alphabetical list of common illnesses and accidents which can be treated by carefully following the guidelines given in the book.

Under each heading there is a description of the illness or accident, followed by a brief outline of some of the most frequently indicated remedies for that disorder.

Each remedy name is followed by a number, which refers to its strength or potency.

The potency number is of great importance when buying remedies and can sometimes be found in minute print on the back of the container.

Choose the remedy that most closely fits the person's physical symptoms, also taking into account any particular emotional or mental pointers. Next, turn to the A–Z of Remedies (pages 50–83) and read the details given there for each remedy before making a final decision. Then refer to instructions given in the Dosage Table on page 12, which indicate the potency to use and how often to repeat the dose.

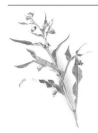
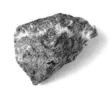
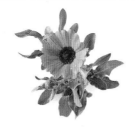
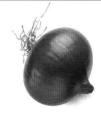
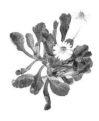

Abortion

Homeopathy can be of great help where a decision to terminate a pregnancy has been taken. Remedies can aid the physical body and also help the mental and emotional state.

CAUTION: Seek immediate professional help if you suspect infection is present after a termination. Signs to watch for are fever, chills, aches and pains in joints and muscles. Any vaginal discharge may change and begin to smell rotten or putrid.

Remedies

Arnica 30 or 200 Reduces the impact of shock to the body. Invaluable to offset the possibility of infection and haemorrhage. Sore, bruised pain.
Bellis Perennis 6 or 30 Use after Arnica (see above). Sore, bruised pain. Mechanical trauma to the womb.
Calendula 6 or 30 This remedy is known as the homeopathic antiseptic, so it may be used where infection is developing, or healing is taking longer than expected. Prevents pus from forming in the blood.
Calendula mother tincture This is very soothing when used to bathe the vaginal area. Soak a sponge in a dilution of 5–10 drops in 300 ml/¹/₂ pint/ 1¹/₄ cups of warm water or use neat.
Ignatia 30 or 200 This is a major remedy for sadness (*see* Sadness).
Pyrogen 30 or 200 For severe septic conditions (*see* Surgery).
Secale 30 or 200 Has not been well since having a termination.
Staphysagria 30 or 200 Take this remedy where there has been surgical intervention or vaginal examination,

particularly if there are feelings of humiliation afterwards (*see* Surgery). The characteristic pain is sharp, stinging, smarting, as if cut.

Abrasions

See *Cuts*.

Abscesses, Boils and Carbuncles

Abscess: A localized collection of pus with redness, swelling and pain. The body's natural response is to wall off the infected area, thus preventing it from spreading to surrounding healthy tissue. Boil: A small area of inflammation which begins in a sweat or fat gland and in the roots of hairs. Carbuncle: A collection of several boils in close proximity. The infection penetrates more deeply than a boil.

CAUTION: Always seek professional help if fever is present.

Remedies

Apis 6 or 30 Stinging, burning pain which is worse for heat in any form, and better for cold applications. The area looks puffy and shiny. The person wants cool air and may be unusually thirstless.
Arnica 6 or 30 Abscesses that do not mature. Crops of boils with bluish area around them. Fear of being touched because of extreme soreness.
Arsenicum 6 or 30 Burning, stabbing pain which feels better for warmth. The person is very restless and anxious.

Belladonna 6 or 30 Threatening abscess with throbbing pain before pus fully develops. Localized heat and redness. The person is very sensitive to touch and light.
Calc Sulph 6x Use after any of the above remedies when thick yellow pus is discharging and shows no sign of abating.
Hepar Sulph 6 or 30 Sharp stabbing pain like a splinter. The person is irritable and extremely sensitive to touch and the slightest draught – must keep warmly wrapped up. Abscess in the armpits (axillae).
Pyrogen 30 or 200 (*See* Surgery).
Silica 6 or 30 Where inflammation and healing take place slowly, this remedy will ripen the boil and help the pus to come out. The area may remain hard long afterwards. There may be abscess of the joints.
CAUTION: This remedy has a centrifugal action which can bring foreign bodies such as splinters to the surface. Caution is essential where there have been implants of any kind in the body.

See also Crotalus Horridus, Ferrum Phos, Lachesis, Tarentula.

Accidents and Emergencies

This section is a general guide. For more detailed information, see also Backache and Back Injuries, Bites and Stings, Bone Injuries and Fractures, Bruises, Burns, Cuts and Abrasions, Eye Injuries, Head Injuries, Haemorrhage, Puncture Wounds, Shock and Collapse, Sprains and

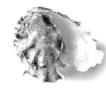 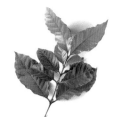 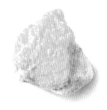 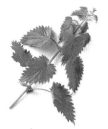 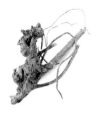

Strains. As well as helping minor injuries, homeopathic remedies can be life-saving in serious situations, while you wait for the ambulance. Give 1 dose of Arnica as fast as you can, as this can reduce haemorrhage, shock and bruising. Arnica is a life-saving plant with a wide range of applications when used in homeopathic dilution. It is the number one accident and emergency remedy.

1 Don't panic!
2 Breathe more deeply.
3 Give Arnica or Rescue Remedy to injured person.
4 Take Arnica or Rescue Remedy yourself.

CAUTION: If the person is unconscious, crush the Arnica between two spoons and drop the powder inside the lip. Alternatively hold one pill just inside the person's lips so that it touches the mucous membrane of the mouth.

Remedies

Arnica 6 or 30 For minor injuries.
Arnica 200 For more serious situations.
Rescue Remedy (Bach Flower Remedies) For any shock or accident situation. Put a few drops on the person's lips, wrists or behind their ears. Repeat frequently. Don't forget to take some yourself.

Acne

This skin condition is usually caused by abnormal activity of fat glands at puberty. Sebaceous ducts become blocked, and blackheads form which turn into pustules if they become infected. The following remedies will help blood cleansing; if the situation persists consult a homeopathic practitioner for deeper treatment.

Remedies

Calc Sulph 6x This helps remove waste products from the blood. Pimples with yellow pus.
Kali Mur 6x For sluggish conditions which are worse after eating fatty or rich food. Skin worse around menstrual period.

Calc Sulph and Kali Mur complement each other and may be used in alternation, e.g. Calc Sulph 6× in the morning and Kali Mur 6× at bedtime for 2 weeks. Repeat after 2 weeks if necessary.

Allergies

See Bites and Stings, Nettle Rash.

Anxiety

See Fear.

Appetite

Eating disorders can arise because of disturbances on all levels – physical, emotional and mental. It is common for appetite to be lost when a person suffers shock or grief, or where there are illnesses with fever, or coughs and colds. Some people reluctant to face problems may stop eating and become anorexic, and food can also be used to suppress emotions by bingeing. Appetite may increase if worms are present. Always seek professional help if the situation becomes prolonged. (See also Constipation, Diarrhoea, Indigestion, Nausea and Vomiting.)

Remedies

Avena Sativa mother tincture A tonic for nervous exhaustion. Stimulates appetite. Dilute 5 drops in water, and take 3 times daily for 2–4 weeks.
Calc Phos 6x Assists digestion and assimilation of food, especially during convalescence. Appetite returns after thinking of food. Can be given to babies who want to feed constantly.
China 6 This remedy has many eating disorders in its symptom picture. There may be aversion to all food; feels full up after even the smallest snack. Hunger without appetite, or ravenous hunger. Hunger after meals.

Arthritis

See Joints.

Asthma

This begins with spasms of the involuntary muscles around the air tubes (bronchi) in the lungs. Mucus collects in these passages, which narrow when the mucous membrane lining swells. The outflow of air is particularly restricted, leading to shortness of breath and wheezing. The many contributory factors include allergies, infection and emotional upsets. There is much discussion over possible links between asthma and childhood inoculations, and asthma which develops after childhood skin eruptions are treated with medicated ointments. It is important to drink frequently to replace the fluids that are lost through rapid breathing. To help relaxation, try a combination of massage and breathing exercises.

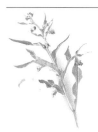
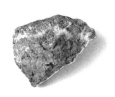
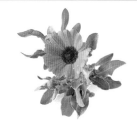
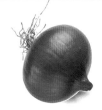
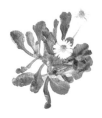

Also try eliminating all dairy and wheat products. Sesame seeds are an alternative source of calcium; these can be bought creamed as tahini, and many foods contain soya, a rich source of protein. Remedies given here may help during acute episodes but a qualified practitioner should always be consulted where there are breathing difficulties. (See also Bronchitis, Coughs, Croup, Whooping Cough.)

Remedies

Arsenicum 6 or 30 Anxious, tosses and turns until they become weak. Worse around midnight.

Bryonia 6 or 30 Wheezing with dryness and not much phlegm. Worse for movement of any kind. Usually irritable.

Chamomilla 6 or 30 Asthma which comes on after anger.

Kali Carb 6 or 30 Breathing difficulties which are relieved by bending forward. Whistling, wheezing; choking cough.

Mag Phos 6x Spasmodic nervous asthma with exhaustion.

Nux Vomica 6 or 30 Asthma linked to stomach disorders. Belching gives some relief. Clothes feel too tight. Finds fault constantly. Angry and impatient.

Pulsatilla 6 or 30 Worse in the evening, in a warm room, and after eating rich or fatty foods. Desires fresh air. May be tearful and clingy.

Athlete's Foot

A skin eruption usually between the toes, attributed to a fungus. Keep the toes dry, and expose to the air as often as possible. As any skin complaint is best treated in a holistic way, it is advisable to consult a homeopath for maximum benefit. However, the following may give relief.

Remedies

Calendula mother tincture Dilute 5–10 drops in a bowl of water and soak feet.

Hepar Sulph 6 or 30 Where there are deep cracks that give off an offensive smell like old cheese.

Silica 6 or 30 Cracks. Acrid, smelly sweat.

Backache and Back Injuries

Backache can be brought on by bad posture, overstraining, sports injuries, kidney infection, womb disorders and spinal anaesthetics in childbirth. Muscles may also tense up when we feel overburdened and then lead to pain. As well as using relevant homeopathic remedies, bodywork is recommended. (See also Accidents and Emergencies.)

Remedies

Arnica 6 or 30 Backache resulting from injury or overstraining. Bruised sore pain.

Arnica mother tincture Add a few drops to bathwater to soothe aches and pains.

Bellis Perennis 6 or 30 Use after Arnica if Arnica does not relieve. Useful after gardening, or occupations with much bending.

Bryonia 6 or 30 Lumbago. Stitching pain and stiffness in the small of the back. Worse from any movement. Better from pressure.

Hypericum 6 or 30 Injuries to the spine, especially the tailbone (coccyx). Pains may shoot along nerve pathways. Useful in childbirth, especially after a forceps delivery.

Kali Carb 6 or 30 Weakness in small of back as if broken. Sudden sharp pain up and down back and thighs. Useful in childbirth when contractions are felt mostly in the back and thighs. Must lie down, or gets relief from bending forward, and from hard pressure.

Mag Phos 6x Neuralgic pains shoot like lightning. Better from warmth, pressure and bending double.

Rhus Tox 6 or 30 Muscular stiffness from overstraining or from exposure to cold, wet weather. Pain on initial movement, feels better once gets going.

Ruta 6 or 30 Sciatica, worse lying at night. Pain extends from back to hips and thighs.

Bedwetting and Incontinence

Normally around the age of three or four, a child will have gained bladder control at night. Where this has not happened and parents are concerned, a patient, positive approach will be most beneficial. There may be irritation in the bladder, or perhaps

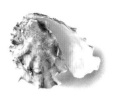 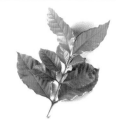  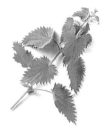 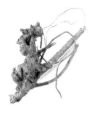

irritation on an emotional level; for example, the child may be feeling jealous of a new brother or sister. In adults incontinence may be caused by weakness of muscles after childbearing or surgery. Constitutional homeopathic treatment is recommended.

Remedies

Causticum 6 or 30 Works well on the muscles of the bladder where urine is lost on coughing, laughing or sneezing. Children wet the bed soon after falling asleep. There may be fear about going to bed alone.

Equisetum 6 or 30 Use where bedwetting seems to have become a habit.

Sepia 6 or 30 Bedwetting soon after falling asleep. Involuntary urination on coughing, sneezing, laughing. Emotionally aloof people who prefer to be alone and dislike fuss.

Bereavement

See *Sadness*.

Bites and Stings

Bites and stings may be painful in varying degrees. After a severe bite or sting from an animal or insect, take one dose of Ledum 6 or 30 immediately. Then select one of the following remedies if necessary.

Remedies

Bee, Wasp, Hornet Stings: Apis, Arnica, Cantharis, Carbolic Acid, Hypericum, Ledum, Urtica Urens.
Externally: Mother tincture of Ledum or Urtica Urens.

Dog, Cat, Horse, Rat Bites: Arnica, Belladonna, Echinacea, Hypericum, Ledum.
Externally: Mother tincture of Hypercal or Ledum.

Gnat, Horsefly, Mosquito Bites: Apis, Cantharis, Hypericum, Ledum.
Externally: Mother tincture of Hypercal or Ledum.

Jellyfish Stings: Apis, Arnica, Hypericum, Ledum, Medusa.
Externally: Mother tincture of Hypercal or Ledum.

Scorpion, Snake, Spider Bites: Arnica, Carbolic Acid, Crotalus Horridus, Echinacea, Lachesis, Ledum.
Externally: Mother tincture of Hypercal or Ledum.

Guiding symptoms for remedies:
Aconite 6 or 30 Shock. Fears will die.
Apis 6 or 30 For any insect bite where there is burning, stinging pain, with a rosy red puffy swelling which is worse for warm and better for cold applications. Give one dose of 200 where there is severe allergic reaction and possible collapse.
Arnica 6 or 30 For shock. Much worse for touch.
Belladonna 30 or 200 Bite from a mad dog. 30th potency: one 2 times daily for 5 days or one dose only of 200. Follow with Lyssin 30 (also called Hydrophobinum): one dose weekly for 4–6 weeks.
Cantharis 6 or 30 Violent burning and smarting pain causing mental excitement. Blisters may develop.

Carbolic Acid 30 or 200 Severe allergic reaction; collapse. Increased sensitivity to smells. Pricking, burning pains. Dusky red face, pale around nose and mouth.
Crotalus Horridus 30 or 200 Rapid deterioration into septic state. Deathly sickness, trembling and exhaustion. Swelling may be bluish, or any colour.
Echinacea mother tincture Blood poisoning; septic states with foul-smelling discharges after animal bites, poisoned wounds. *Internally:* dilute 5 drops in $^1/_4$ glass of water, 3 times daily for 1 week.
Hypericum 6 or 30 Very severe pain which shoots along nerve pathways from injury. Can prevent tetanus from developing.
Lachesis 6 or 30 Purplish-blue skin around bite. Much worse from the slightest touch. Intolerant to pressure of clothes.
Ledum 6 or 30 Prevents tetanus. For any puncture wound where the part feels cold and is better for cold applications. Watery swelling which may be red and inflamed.
Medusa 6 or 30 Numbness and burning pricking heat, especially after jellyfish stings.
Staphysagria 6 or 30 Large bites which itch violently, with smarting, stinging pain.
Urtica Urens 6 or 30 Stinging burning pains.

CAUTION: Always seek immediate professional help in any serious situation.

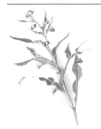
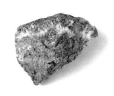
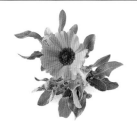
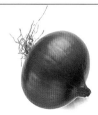
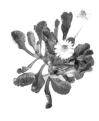

Bleeding

See *Accidents and Emergencies, Dentist, Haemorrhage, Nosebleeds, Surgery.*

Blood Poisoning

Blood poisoning, or septicaemia, is a serious condition. Bacteria may enter the bloodstream from an infected wound and spread throughout the body. Symptoms to watch for are fever together with joint and muscle pain, sweating, shivering and possible abscess. Seek urgent medical help; meanwhile, choose one of the following remedies. (See also Abscesses, Bites and Stings.)

Remedies

Baptisia 30 or 200 Very important remedy for smouldering fevers. Heavy, sore, aching muscles. Restless and confused. Dark red face and mucous membranes. Tongue may feel burnt.

Echinacea mother tincture This is a natural antibiotic. Aching limbs, weakness, slowness. Blood poisoning from insect stings, snake bites and poisonous plants. Useful when travelling. Dilute 5 drops in ¼ glass of water and take 3 times daily for 1 week.

Pyrogen 30 or 200 Bruised, sore, aching pain. Restless. Rosy-red streaks from wounds. Chronic complaints that date back to septic conditions.

Secale 30 or 200 Numbness, tingling, pricking pains. Internal burning heat but feels icy-cold externally, refuses to be covered.

Bone Injuries and Fractures

If it is necessary to move the person before other help arrives, make a splint to prevent movement of the injured part. Treat for shock, and after bones have been set, begin giving either Calc Phos or Symphytum or give them in alternation for 7–10 days.

Remedies

Arnica 30 or 200 For shock and bruised sore pain. Swellings with discoloration.

Bryonia 6 or 30 Especially for fractured ribs. Worse for any movement. May be irritable.

Calc Phos 6x Because it affects the nutrition of bones and promotes ossification, this remedy will help fractures to heal much faster. Use only when you know the bone has been set properly. Can be used in alternation with Symphytum.

Eupatorium Perf 6 or 30 Violent aching pain in bones.

Hypericum 30 or 200 Severe pain shooting along nerve pathways.

Ledum 6 or 30 Where swelling remains after Arnica has been given. The part feels cold to the touch and yet is better for cold applications.

Ruta 6 or 30 Injuries to the covering of bones (periosteum), particularly the shin bones. Fractures of wrist (Colles') or ankles (Potts'). Bruised sore pain.

Symphytum 6x The common names of this plant are Knitbone or Boneset, which illustrate clearly its use. Use this remedy only after the part has been positioned correctly in a plaster cast, as it promotes fast healing of bone. Swellings with no discoloration.

Symphytum can be used in alternation with Calc Phos.

CAUTION: Only use Calc Phos and Symphytum when you know that bones have been set in the correct position. Do not use if a pin has been inserted.

Breastfeeding and Mastitis

If a newborn baby suckles immediately after birth, this will not only stimulate milk to flow, but also help the uterus to contract. Homeopathic remedies can be used to help increase or decrease the amount of milk, or to dry it up.

Remedies
Milk Flow

Lac Caninum 6 or 30 This remedy will encourage the milk flow to increase. It may also be used to dry it up where the woman decides to discontinue breastfeeding, or where there has been a stillbirth, or the baby has died. A characteristic of this remedy is that physical symptoms may move back and forth from one breast to the other.

Pulsatilla 6 or 30 Used in the same way as Lac Can for the flow of milk. In addition, the person who needs this remedy is tearful and feels better for being comforted. She desires fresh air and feels worse in a warm room.

Urtica Urens 6 or 30 This remedy can also increase or arrest the flow of milk. There may be burning, stinging pain in the breasts.

Cracked Nipples

Calendula ointment and Calendula mother tincture Use the ointment

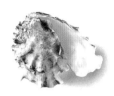
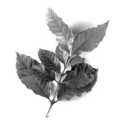
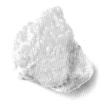
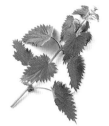
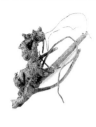

liberally before and after baby is born to soften nipples. Once cracks appear, bathe nipples in diluted Calendula mother tincture, and apply Calendula ointment. This will soothe and speed up healing. If persistent, use one of the following:

Castor Equi 6 or 30 Cracked or ulcerated nipples. Much worse for touch of clothing.

Hepar Sulph 6 or 30 Cracks with pus in them. May smell like old cheese. The person is irritable and very sensitive to draughts.

Silica 6 or 30 Sharp pains when baby nurses.

Mastitis

Breasts inflame usually because of bacterial infection from a cracked nipple, and an abscess may form. The breast gets congested, hard, hot and painful, and may be red.

Belladonna 30 or 200 High fever. Extremely painful engorgement, much worse for the slightest jarring or touch. Breast is red or may have red streaks. There may be a throbbing or bursting headache, with much sensitivity to light. Symptoms develop suddenly.

Bryonia 30 or 200 The onset is slower than with Belladonna. Stony hard swelling where the person may prefer to lie on the painful breast to keep it still because all movement aggravates.

Phytolacca 30 or 200 Breasts have stony hard lumps. Cracked nipples are sore and tender. When the baby feeds, the pains radiate over the whole body.

Bronchitis

An inflammation and infection of the bronchial passages in the lungs, with fever. A cough ensues with pain and tightness behind the breastbone (sternum). Breathing becomes faster than usual. Symptoms of acute bronchitis may develop when a cold settles on the chest, or after exposure to cold damp weather, or dusty, smoky environment. It may also accompany childhood infectious disorders such as whooping cough and measles (see Asthma, Coughs, Croup, Measles, Whooping Cough). Inhaling steam may be helpful but DO NOT use products with menthol, eucalyptus or peppermint (e.g. Friars Balsam, Vick's VapoRub, etc.) as these may prevent remedies from working (see Antidotes, page 12).

Remedies

Aconite 6 or 30 Feverish colds and coughs which come on suddenly after exposure to very cold dry winds. Aconite may prevent illness developing further if taken in the early stages. There may be fear and restlessness.

Ant Tart 6 or 30 Loose, rattling cough with chest full of phlegm, which becomes more and more difficult to raise because of weakness. Worse from warm drinks.

Bryonia 6 or 30 Dry, very painful cough with stitching pain. Holds chest during cough to prevent movement, or lies on the painful side. The cough is worse while eating or drinking. Irritability may be present, with a desire to be left alone.

Ferrum Phos 6x Useful if taken in the very early stages of feverish conditions.

Hepar Sulph 6 or 30 Cough and loss of voice after being in cold dry wind. Weakness and rattling in chest, difficulty raising the phlegm, which is thick yellow. Child cries before coughing. Barking, choking cough, worse from cold drinks (Ant Tart is worse from warm drinks). Worse from the slightest uncovering.

Phosphorus 6 or 30 People who need Phosphorus may appear well when ill. Cough with burning, tightness and a feeling of a weight in the chest. Cough is worse for talking, laughing and breathing cold air. Rust-coloured sputum. There may be thirst for ice-cold water which aggravates the cough. Better for company. Fear when alone.

Pulsatilla 6 or 30 Cough worse in a heated room, better outdoors. A sense of heaviness in the chest. Loose cough in the morning, dry in the evening. Must sit up in bed at night to cough. Child may cry or whine and won't let you disappear from sight.

Sulphur 6 or 30 Wants windows open. Burning or coldness in chest. Weakness in chest while talking. Very sleepy in the day, wakeful at night. Redness of lips, and ears. This remedy is often indicated at the end of an acute illness where progress comes to a standstill.

Bruises

When the body is bruised, blood seeps from damaged vessels into surrounding tissue and turns blue as it decomposes. The most commonly used remedy for bruising is Arnica, which can be used externally in the form of ointment or mother tincture,

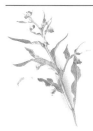
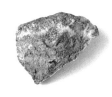
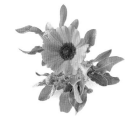
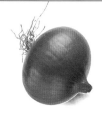
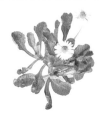

as well as in tablet form. (See also *Bone Injuries and Fractures.*)

CAUTION: Never use Arnica externally on any area where the skin is broken as it can cause a rash.

Remedies

Arnica 6 or 30 Bruised muscles and connective tissue. Rapidly aids absorption of effused blood. Swellings which accompany bruising usually reduce very quickly with Arnica but if there is little reaction, use Ledum.

Hypericum 6 or 30 Bruised nerves. Use where there is sharp shooting pain in punctured or penetrating wounds. Painful scars. Prevents tetanus.

Ledum 6 or 30 Helps blood reabsorption. May be needed if swelling remains after taking Arnica. Affected parts are cold and worse for warmth.

Ruta 6 or 30 Bruises to coverings of bones (periosteum), particularly shinbones.

Bunions

A bunion is a deformity of the joint at the base of the big toe which may occasionally become inflamed and painful.

Remedies

Agaricus 6 or 30 Pain as if pierced by needles, with ice-cold tingling and numbness.

Ruta 6 or 30 Pain worse in cold wet weather. Use Ruta ointment externally.

Burns

*Burns have three main categories: **1st degree:** The skin becomes red only. **2nd degree:** The burn begins to destroy living tissue; blisters develop. **3rd degree:** The burns are deep and involve all layers of skin. These can become life-threatening. Dangers with burns are shock, loss of body fluids and that sepsis may develop. Much can be done to reduce pain, shock and prevent sepsis with homeopathic remedies, but **in serious cases act swiftly by calling an ambulance immediately**. The degree of danger to life depends not so much on the depth of the burn, but on how large the damaged area is.*

Remedies for Serious Burns

Counteract shock and prevent person from becoming too cold. Relieve pain by giving one of the following remedies. Repeat when the pain begins to return.

Aconite 30 or 200 For fear and shock with much restlessness.

Arnica 30 or 200 For shock. May deny anything is wrong.

Cantharis 30 or 200 For the pain.

Causticum 6 or 30 To relieve pain of deep burns.

Externally: Immediately place burnt area under running cold water to help reduce pain and swelling. Don't tear off clothing as this may pull skin with it. Cover any exposed area with a dressing and soak in **Hypercal mother tincture** 5–10 drops to 300 ml/½ pint/1¼ cups of cool water, preferably water that has previously been boiled. Continue soaking the dressing as it dries out.

Calendula ointment can be applied to the edges of the burn.

Remedies for Minor Burns

Urtica Urens 6 or 30 To relieve pain.

Calendula mother tincture 5 drops in water for scalded mouth.

Caesarean Section

See *Surgery.*

Carbuncles

See *Abscesses.*

Catarrh and Sinusitis

Inflammation of a mucous membrane with excessive formation of mucus. The term 'catarrh' is normally used in relation to the nose and throat, and 'sinusitis' refers to inflammation of the sinuses, which are a continuation of the nose cavity.

Remedies

Bryonia 6 or 30 Catarrh extends from nose to sinuses or chest. Mucous membranes feel dry. Bursting, splitting headaches. Better outdoors on damp, cloudy days.

Hepar Sulph 6 or 30 Thick, yellow, offensive catarrh with pain and swelling of nose, and hoarseness. Feels irritable and worse for slightest draught.

Kali Bic 6 or 30 Thick, stringy green or yellow mucus. Pressure or stuffed-up feeling at the root of the nose. Chronic inflammation of frontal sinuses. Violent sneezing in the morning.

Kali Mur 6x Stuffy cold in head. Thick white discharge. Worse in open air.

Kali Sulph 6x Yellow, slimy discharges.

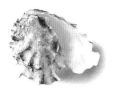
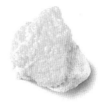
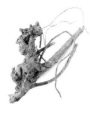
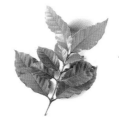
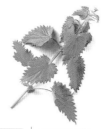

Worse in the evening and in a warm room, better in open air.

Nat Mur 6x Frequent sneezing with gushing of clear watery or thick white discharge which tastes salty or bitter. May be worse on alternate days.

Pulsatilla 6 or 30 Bland, thick yellow mucus. Nose stuffs up at night and indoors; discharges freely in open air. Feels better sitting up in bed. Loss of smell.

Chest

See *Asthma, Bronchitis, Coughs, Whooping Cough.*

Chickenpox

Chickenpox is an infectious illness of childhood, but may sometimes occur in adulthood. A bout normally gives life-long immunity. There is an incubation period of 10–21 days after which an itchy rash appears, with or without a fever. The spots are small, red and raised and become inflamed blisters, which may contain pus. When they burst, scabs develop, and if scratched will form scars. The rash usually appears first on the back and chest, then on the face, arms and legs. It is contagious from the day before the rash appears until the last scab has dropped off.

Remedies

Aconite 6 or 30 In the early stages. High fever with restlessness and anxiety.

Ant Tart 6 or 30 The rash develops slowly; there may be a coarse, rattling cough or bronchitis.

Belladonna 6 or 30 High fever, flushed face, inability to sleep.

Pulsatilla 6 or 30 A whining, weepy child who won't be left alone. There may be very little or no thirst, even with fever.

Rhus Tox 6 or 30 The main remedy for chickenpox. All symptoms worse at night. Restless sleep. Sensitive to cold air.

Chilblains

These occur in toes, fingers and ears when there is a sluggish circulation which is made worse by cold weather. Local blood vessels become engorged, and redness, itching and burning ensue, sometimes with cracking of the skin.

Remedies

Agaricus 6 or 30 Pain as if pierced by cold or hot needles. Skin feels frozen. Improves circulation by bringing elasticity back to blood vessels. Cracked skin.

Ferrum Phos 6x Where there is redness, heat and swelling.

Pulsatilla 6 or 30 Itching is worse in a warm room.

Externally: **Tamus ointment** or **Calendula ointment.**

Cold Sores

The Herpes simplex virus is often carried throughout life and may surface if the person is in a lowered state of vitality. Inflamed blisters appear, usually around the mouth or lips, and sometimes on nostrils, eyes or genitals. Constitutional treatment is recommended.

Remedies

Arsenicum 6 or 30 Eruptions on lips with burning, stinging pain.

Hepar Sulph 6 or 30 Pus forms. Sores are very much worse for touch. Person is cold and irritable.

Nat Mur 6x Sores of watery blisters on the lips or at the edge of the hair. They may appear with a cold. Lips are cracked.

Colds

A cold is an acute inflammation of the mucous membranes of the nose and throat. It is the body's attempt to throw off unwanted matter. For this reason, it can be detrimental to health to cut short a cold with large doses of Vitamin C because what was attempting to find an exit route is then added to the body's toxic load.

The remedies mentioned here may help with the acute stage, but if you are prone to frequent colds, constitutional homeopathic treatment can help strengthen your immune system so that you become less susceptible to them. (See also Coughs, Fevers.)

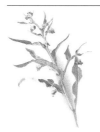
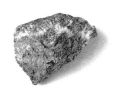
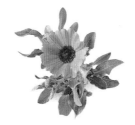
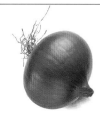
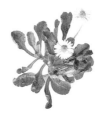

Remedies

Aconite 6 or 30 Colds that come on suddenly after being out in harsh winds. Frequent sneezing and watery discharge which may be hot.

Arsenicum 6 or 30 Burning, water discharge. Much sneezing. Restless. Anxious. Can't get warm enough.

Bryonia 6 or 30 Colds, which may descend to chest, begin with sneezing. Bursting headache. Feels better alone and in cool, open air.

Dulcamara 6 or 30 Chills come after sudden exposure to cold, wet weather, especially after being heated (e.g. in summer and autumn).

Eupatorium Perf 6 or 30 Flu-like symptoms. Severe aching, soreness in bones. Sore eyeballs. Chills preceded by thirst.

Gelsemium 6 or 30 Typical flu or summer colds. Chills up and down back. Drowsiness. Heaviness. Thirstless.

Nat Mur 6x Begins with sneezing. Nose drips water, or thick white discharge. Loss of taste and smell.

Nux Vomica 6 or 30 A chilly person. Nose blocked at night, runs in the morning, may be one side only. Nose itches. Symptoms better in cold air, worse in warm room.

Colic

Powerful contraction or spasm of involuntary muscle in the abdomen. It is a symptom of inflammation or obstruction, or may be brought on in breastfed babies by the mother eating acidic fruit or highly seasoned food, and can cause much distress. Anger can be another cause, and in adults gallstones may be present.

Remedies

Chamomilla 6 or 30 Person tosses about in despair. Nothing pleases, and bad-tempered babies are passed from one person to another in an effort to pacify them.

Colocynth 6 or 30 Violent cutting pain. This remedy is often indicated when the cause is anger. Better for hard pressure on the abdomen and for bending double. Babies get relief from being placed on the stomach.

Dioscorea 6 or 30 Unbearable sharp, cutting, twisting pain that radiates to distant parts. Some relief from stretching out or bending backwards.

Mag Phos 6x Spasms of cramp which are relieved by warmth and gentle massage.

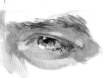

Staphysagria 6 or 30 Colic in a child after being reprimanded, or after anger. Flatus smells like rotten eggs.

Concentration

Poor concentration and memory loss have innumerable causes. Remedies given here will help where there is mental strain from overwork or overstudying.

Remedies

Aethusa 6 Weakness and inability to think or focus from overstudying. Difficulty in holding the head up. Goes into examination and can remember nothing.

Anacardium 6 Nervous exhaustion from overstudy. Poor memory. Low self-confidence.

Calc Phos 6x Mental strain from overstudying. Useful at puberty.

Anxious about the future. Alternate with Kali Phos 6x.

Kali Phox 6x Poor memory in students. Irritable and nervous. Sleeplessness from worrying.

Concussion

See *Head Injuries*.

Confidence

See *Fear and Anxiety*.

Conjunctivitis

Inflammation of the membrane covering the eyeball and under the lids, causing the eye to become bloodshot and itch, with a gritty feeling. One or both eyes may be affected. Discharge is thin and watery or thick and sticky. Light sensitivity (photophobia) may be present. (See also Eye Injuries, Eyestrain, Styes.)

Remedies

Apis 6 or 30 Eyelids are swollen and puffy. Pains burn and sting, and the person feels better in cool air.

Belladonna 6 or 30 Heat, redness and throbbing pain. Sensitive to light.

Euphrasia 6 or 30 Watery or sticky acrid discharge from eyes, bland nasal discharge. Occurs with measles.

Euphrasia mother tincture Dilute two drops in cooled, boiled water in an eyebath.

Pulsatilla 6 or 30 Comes on with a cold. Thick yellowy-green discharge. Person feels better in open air.

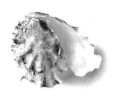
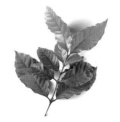
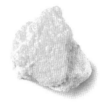
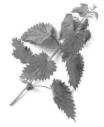
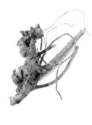

Constipation

This is a state of the bowels in which irregular evacuations are hard and expelled with difficulty. Purging with laxatives irritates the intestine and can create a habit whereby the body forgets what it is supposed to do. Fresh vegetables, whole grains and some fruit contain plenty of roughage which, along with regular exercise, will help a sluggish bowel to become more active. Large quantities of bran should not be necessary. However, if constipation persists, seek professional help as it may be the result of a deep-seated tendency to 'hold on' or indicative of a more serious disorder.

Remedies

Bryonia 6 or 30 Chronic constipation with bursting headaches. Stools are large and hard, and dry as if burnt. Irritable, thirsty person.

Kali Mur 6x Light-coloured stools. White-coated tongue. Fats and pastries disagree.

Lycopodium 6 or 30 Constipated when away from home. Noisy flatulence. Feels worse from pressure of clothes. Irritable in the morning, on waking.

Nat Mur 6x Dry, hard stools. Watery secretions from other areas such as the eyes. May be retention of stools on alternate days. Craves salty food.

Nux Vomica 6 or 30 Unsatisfactory urging with feeling of incomplete evacuation. Worse while travelling or wearing tight clothes around waist. People who lead sedentary lives.

Sepia 6 or 30 Sensation of a lump remaining in rectum after stool. Feels sluggish, and dragged down in mind and body. Constipation during menses or in pregnancy.

Silica 6 or 30 Stool recedes after being partly expelled because of weakness, or person holds on to stool through fear of pain.

Corns

A cone or horn of dead tissue forms in the outer layer of skin and may be caused by wearing badly-fitting shoes. A homeopath would look for the tendency to develop callosities (or hardness) in other areas.

Remedies

Ant Crud 6 or 30 Thick, hard callosities on soles of feet which are extremely tender to walk on.

Arnica 6 or 30 For bruised, sore pain.

Externally: **Arnica mother tincture.**

Calc Fluor 6x Thickened skin which cracks and becomes hard.

Ferrum Phos 6x Pain with heat and throbbing.

Silica 6x Soft corns between toes. Cold sweat on feet which may smell offensive and destroy shoes.

Coughs

Coughing is a reflex action produced by the stimulation of nerve endings. It rids air passages of unwanted debris, including mucus produced during infections of the lungs. Having a cough, therefore, is not necessarily something to be banished as soon as it appears, since its main function is to keep the lungs in a healthier condition. Coughing may also be connected to sadness or deep disappointment. (See also Asthma, Bronchitis, Croup, Whooping Cough).

Remedies

Aconite 6 or 30 Short, dry cough, which comes on suddenly after exposure to cold, dry, windy weather. There may be anxiety and restlessness.

Belladonna 6 or 30 Child may cry before coughing and go red in the face. Dry, barking cough with headache, as if head will burst. Cough ends with sneezing.

Bryonia 6 or 30 Dry, hard cough, worse on entering a warm room. Stitching pain in chest, worse for any movement so holds chest when coughing. Feels better on cloudy, damp days. Irritable and prefers to be left alone.

Causticum 6 or 30 Cannot cough deep enough because of weakness of muscles; phlegm slips back. Tight chest. Tickling in throat, better for sips of cold water. Urine escapes on coughing. Shortness of breath while talking.

Rumex 6 or 30 Dry, teasing cough, like tickling from a feather. Much worse from breathing cold air, or sudden change from a warm to a cold room, or cold to warm. Closes or covers the mouth when coughing.

Sulphur 6 or 30 A hot person who prefers doors and windows open. Burning in chest. Cough worse at night, and when having a bath. May have very red lips or ears.

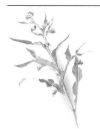
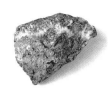
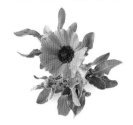
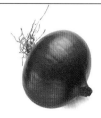
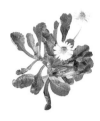

Cramp

See *Pain*.

Croup

Croup is characterized by swelling of the larynx which causes breathing to sound hoarse and croaky. A paroxysmal cough creates a sense of suffocation, with accompanying fear. Croup usually develops in or is made worse by dry weather; for some people steam inhalations can give relief, but DO NOT use things such as Friar's Balsam or Vick's VapoRub as these contain substances which antidote homeopathic remedies (see page 12).

Remedies

Aconite 6 or 30 Sudden onset after exposure to cold, dry winds. A short, barking cough, with feeling of suffocation. Restless and anxious.

Hepar Sulph 6 or 30 Similar to Aconite, with its onset after exposure to cold, dry wind, but this person is irritated or made much worse from the slightest uncovering of any part of the body, even putting a hand out of bed. Rattly chest but cannot bring phlegm up. Child cries before coughing. Cough is worse from cold drinks.

Spongia 6 or 30 Hoarseness with hollow, barking cough which sounds like a saw. Wakes with sense of suffocation and great anxiety (like Aconite). Larynx worse for touch. Better eating and drinking warm things.

Cuts and Abrasions

Remedies can be used for minor cuts and more serious infected wounds. Calendula or Hypercal mother tincture is invaluable in a first-aid kit.

Remedies

Arnica 6 or 30 For any shock, bruising, bleeding. *Externally:* **Calendula mother tincture** Promptly stops bleeding in small wounds and inhibits the growth of harmful bacteria, thus preventing pus formation and infection. Cleanse the wound with a dilution of 5–10 drops in 300ml/ $^1/_2$ pint/$1^1/_4$ cups of water. If a large dressing is being applied, soak lint in this dilution and leave it undisturbed while healing takes place; as it dries out, reapply the diluted tincture.

Calendula ointment can be applied round the edges of or on a wound after it has been cleaned. One of the symptoms of Calendula is that pain is out of proportion to the injury.

Hypercal ointment can be used in the same way as Calendula, and combines the properties of both plants (Calendula and Hypericum). Wounds in Hypericum are more tender than their appearance would indicate.

Cystitis

*Inflammation of the bladder (urinary tract infection), usually from bacteria. Symptoms are frequent, painful urging to pass urine. Bacteria can come from neighbouring organs, be introduced on a catheter after an operation, or develop as a result of sexual activity. Drink cranberry juice, and plenty of water, especially pot barley water, but if it is recurrent, or if there is pain in the lower back with fever, and/or blood in the urine, **seek professional help**.*

Remedies

Apis 6 or 30 Much straining, then a few drops of hot, maybe bloody urine are passed. Agonizing, sharp, burning, stinging pain. Worse from heat, better from being cool. Often thirstless.

Cantharis 6 or 30 Violent, burning, cutting, stabbing pain which is worse before and after urinating. Doubles up. Urine passed drop by drop. Intense pain and excitement.

Causticum 6 or 30 Painful retention after an operation or brought on by cold weather.

Nux Vomica 6 or 30 Painful, ineffectual urging to urinate. A chilly person, often irritable.

Staphysagria 6 or 30 Burning during and after urinating. Useful after operations to female reproductive organs, or where there has been new or frequent sexual activity.

Dandruff

Scaly dead skin which flakes off the scalp in noticeable proportions, often due to over-activity of oil-forming glands. This imbalance responds well to regular treatment from a professional homeopath.

Remedies

Arsenicum 6 or 30 Very sensitive scalp. Skin

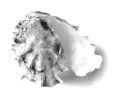 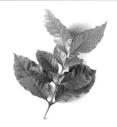  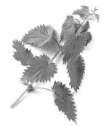 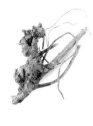

flakes off in white scales. Chilly, irritable, restless person. Anxious about health.
Kali Mur 6x White scales.
Kali Sulph 6x Yellow scales.

Dentist

People sometimes put off visiting the dentist because they find it an ordeal, and children may not want to return after an initial difficult experience. Remedies mentioned here will help with anxiety, and with pain after treatment. (See also Fear and Anxiety, Teething Babies, Toothache.)

Remedies

Aconite 6 or 30 For great fear, panic and restlessness.
Arnica 6 or 30 One before and one immediately after treatment. Helps prepare the body for any shock to the system, as well as being a preventative for haemorrhage and bruising.
Gelsemium 6 or 30 Anxiety which causes frequent emptying of bladder or bowels. Trembling in any part of the body. May help clear unfocused feeling in head after injections.
Hypericum 6 or 30 Extreme pains which shoot along nerve pathway.
Ruta 6 or 30 Pain after tooth extraction, not relieved by Arnica. Pain settles in the jaw bones.
Externally: **Hypercal mother tincture** Use as a mouthwash. Halts bleeding, reduces swelling and prevents sepsis. Dilute 5–10 drops in 150 ml/¼ pint/½ cup of water.

Diarrhoea

*The remedies in this section are for diarrhoea which comes on as a result of food poisoning, or after strong emotional reactions such as fear or shock, and in teething babies. **With severe symptoms in babies and young children, seek professional advice within 24 hours** as dehydration can develop fast; signs are sunken eyes, no saliva or tears, and pinched skin which loses its ability to fall back into place. Offer plenty of drinks. Where diarrhoea is of a more chronic nature, constitutional treatment is recommended. (See also Colic, Fear and Anxiety.)*

Remedies

Aconite 6 or 30 Diarrhoea from fright.
Arg Nit 6 or 30 Noisy diarrhoea, food and drink go straight through, especially worse for sugar. For anticipatory anxiety before an ordeal. Feels worse in a confined space.
Arsenicum 6 or 30 Food poisoning, or diarrhoea after eating watery fruits, or cold foods. Symptoms develop around midnight. There may be intense restlessness, anxiety and weakness.
Chamomilla 6 or 30 Greenish stools smelling of rotten eggs. Babies are very bad-tempered and insist on being carried.
Cuprum 6 or 30 Diarrhoea with intense cramps.
Gelsemium 6 or 30 Painless diarrhoea in nervous people after anticipation of a forthcoming event, or after a sudden fright.
Mag Phos 6 or 30 Severe colicky pain with cramp. Relief comes from doubling up, pressure, and particularly from heat.

Pulsatilla 6 or 30 No two stools look alike. Diarrhoea from eating rich, fatty foods, ices or eggs. Worse in the evening and in a warm room.
Sulphur 6 or 30 Urgency, rushes out of bed in the morning. Anus red, sore and itchy after stools. Always too hot, kicks covers off in bed, or sticks feet out.
Veratrum Alb 6 or 30 Copious evacuations – of vomiting, diarrhoea and cold sweat on forehead. May be simultaneous stools and vomiting. Icy coldness of different parts. Profound weakness or fainting.

Digestion

See *Indigestion.*

Dislocation

See *Sprains.*

Dizziness

See *Vertigo.*

Earache

*Earache is commonly caused by infection spreading up the Eustachian tubes from the nose, throat or sinuses (middle-ear infection, or otitis media). A build-up of pus may create such pressure that the drum bursts, giving an outlet for the pus, with instant relief of pain. **Seek immediate medical attention where there is severe pain, especially if there is redness, swelling and tenderness of bone behind the ear.** Changes in atmospheric pressure (for example, at high altitude) can also cause earache.*

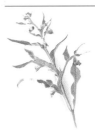
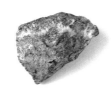
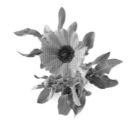
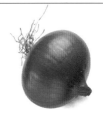
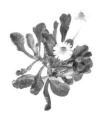

Remedies

Aconite 6 or 30 Sudden onset from cold, dry winds.

Apis 6 or 30 External ear red and inflamed. Screams with pain. Worse in a warm room.

Belladonna 6 or 30 Throbbing pain causing child to cry out in sleep. High fever. Hot head with cold limbs. Delirium. The right ear is more commonly affected.

Chamomilla 6 or 30 Earache may accompany teething. Inconsolable child wants to be carried all the time. Nothing seems to alleviate the pain – except a dose of Chamomilla!

Ferrum Phos 6x For the early stages where there is heat, throbbing and the beginnings of inflammation.

Hepar Sulph 6 or 30 Pain goes from throat to ears on swallowing. Sharp, splinter-like pain. Worse from any draught – covers ear to keep warm.

Kali Mur 6x Deafness from catarrhal condition. Noises in ear on blowing nose. Very useful for pain at high altitude.

Mag Phos 6x Severe sharp pain, worse in cold air; relieved by warmth and pressure.

Pulsatilla 6 or 30 External ear red and swollen. There may be a thick yellow-green discharge, with pain worse from warmth and at night. Child is tearful or whiny, and wants lots of comforting.

Silica 6 or 30 Perforated eardrum. Catarrhal deafness. Shy, timid children, who are sensitive to cold draughts.

Emergencies

See *Accidents.*

Enuresis

See *Bedwetting and Incontinence.*

Episiotomy

See *Labour.*

Exam Nerves

See *Fear and Anxiety.*

Eye Injuries

Seek prompt medical help for serious injuries or if a foreign body becomes lodged in the eye. (See also Eyestrain.)

Remedies

Aconite 6 or 30 To relieve immediate pain and shock.

Arnica 6 or 30 For bruising to soft tissue around eye.

Hypericum 6 or 30 Extremely painful injury, with shooting pains.

Ledum 6 or 30 Injuries which are relieved by cold.

Symphytum 6 or 30 Injury from a blow to the eyeball.

Externally: **Calendula mother tincture** To control bleeding, or to soothe if there has been a foreign body in the eye, dilute 2 drops in an eyebath.

Euphrasia mother tincture Relieves many eye complaints. Dilute 2 drops in an eye bath.

Eyestrain

Brought on by excessive work at a computer keyboard, or from other close work such as reading or sewing.

Remedies

Euphrasia 6 or 30 Red, burning, watery eyes. Abundant hot tears creating soreness.

Ruta 6 or 30 Eyes are hot, red and painful. Vision seems dim. Spasm in lower eyelids.

Externally: **Euphrasia mother tincture** 2 drops diluted in an eyebath.

Fainting

Fainting is a result of a temporary reduction in the supply of oxygen to the brain. Bending the head below the knees will reverse this process. Fainting can be caused by excitement, shock, severe pain or prolonged standing.

Remedies

Bryonia 6 or 30 Faints while standing or at every attempt to sit up.

Chamomilla 6 or 30 Faints from extreme pain.

China 6 or 30 Faints from loss of blood or other body fluids.

Coffea 6 or 30 Faints from being over-excited, and in childbirth.

Ignatia 6 or 30 Faints from shock, grief or other emotions. Oversensitive, dramatic people, or those who sit silently brooding.

Nux Vomica 6 or 30 Faints from pain. Also brought on by smells and bright lights.

Phosphorus 6 or 30 Faints from slight causes, from smells, or being hungry.

Pulsatilla 6 or 30 Faints in a warm, stuffy room.

Fear and Anxiety

Fear is an automatic response to

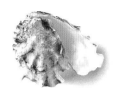
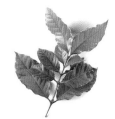

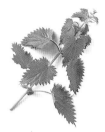
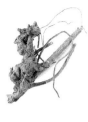

danger or to situations where we feel uncomfortable in some way. The endocrine glands respond by producing extra adrenalin and we become more alert, our hearts beat faster, breathing becomes more rapid and we may sweat.

This could be useful if we were being chased by a tiger, but often reactions are from habit. When fear dominates us, an abnormal load is placed on the physical body because poisons are released into the bloodstream at this time. Early warning signals are digestive disorders, headaches or a rise in blood pressure. If the signals are ignored, chronic ill health may result. Remedies are suggested for helping in some of the more common situations, such as taking an exam or a driving test, or visiting the dentist or hospital.

Remedies

Aconite 6 or 30 Great fear and panic, agitation and restlessness. Fear of death. Useful where fear remains after a shock or difficult experience, but the agitation may not be shown.

Arg Nit 6 or 30 Nervous. Impulsive and hurried. Timid. Fear in confined spaces or looking down from a height. Diarrhoea brought on by fear and anxiety. Better in cool, open air.

Gelsemium 6 or 30 Feeling of anticipation and dread before an event. Trembling and weakness of limbs. Heaviness anywhere. Increased urination or nervous painless diarrhoea. Headache feels better for frequent emptying of bladder. Confusion and sleepiness.

Ignatia 6 or 30 Oversensitive, highly emotional with dramatic mood swings. May sigh a lot.

Kali Phos 6x This beneficially soothes and calms the nervous system. Sleepless from anxiety. A few doses hourly before bed can aid sleep.

Lycopodium 6 or 30 Social situations cause anxiety, but insecurity and lack of confidence may be hidden behind an act of bravado. Indecisive and timid. Much rumbling and flatulence in abdomen. Symptoms worse between 4 p.m. and 8 p.m.

Mag Phos 6x Muscle cramps and trembling from nervous tension. Sharp neuralgic pains which are relieved by heat and by bending double.

Silica 6 or 30 Lack of 'grit'. Shy, timid person, often feels chilly.

Fever

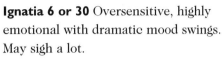

A fever is the body's response to certain illnesses and is to be welcomed as an attempt to restore normal balance. If fever is suppressed, it weakens the efforts of the immune system. Give plenty of fluids, and cool down by sponging small areas with tepid water. If fever continues to rise very high, seek medical help. (See also *Blood Poisoning*.)

Remedies

Aconite 6 or 30 Sudden onset after exposure to dry cold winds. Person maybe very restless and fearful.

Arsenicum 6 or 30 Symptoms come on suddenly. Restless. Relieved by warmth, even though they are hot. Desires frequent sips of water. May become increasingly weak and anxious.

Belladonna 6 or 30 Very high fever, face is fiery red, eyes look glassy and there is very little thirst. May be delirious and moan and toss about during sleep. Dryness everywhere. Eyes are very sensitive to light. Hot head with cold limbs. Throbbing headache.

Bryonia 6 or 30 Feels worse from the slightest movement, even of eyes. Very thirsty for large quantities of water.

Ferrum Phos 6x For the beginnings of fever. Throbbing pains with inflammation of soft parts. Great weakness.

Gelsemium 6 or 30 Flu symptoms. Person aches all over; there may be heaviness anywhere, even of eyelids. Feels cold shivers up and down back. Thirstless.

Phosphorus 6 or 30 Very thirsty for ice-cold drinks. Colds may go to the chest. People who need this remedy often look surprisingly well when they are ill. Hunger with fever.

Pulsatilla 6 or 30 Normally thirstless. Children are tearful, fretful and want lots of cuddles.

Flatulence

See *Indigestion*.

Flu

See *Colds, Coughs, Fever, Throat*.

Food Poisoning

See *Blood Poisoning, Diarrhoea, Nausea and Vomiting*.

31

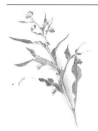
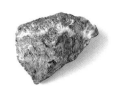
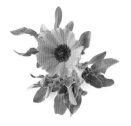
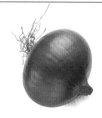
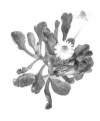

Fractures

See *Bone Injuries*.

Frostbite

*Exposed parts first
lose the sense of
feeling, then turn white,
and later become blue.
Rubbing may cause damage,
but gently patting the area with snow
may help to stimulate the local blood
supply back into action. Gentle
warmth is the most important thing to
provide. Frostbitten areas will be
vulnerable to infection, so wrap the
affected part in a sterile dressing
which has been soaked in Hypercal
mother tincture (5–10 drops to 300 ml/
½ pint/1¼ cups of boiled water).*

Remedies

Agaricus 6 or 30 Burning, itching,
redness and swelling. Legs feel heavy,
as if they do not belong to the person.
They feel as if they have been pierced
by hot or cold needles.

Apis 6 or 30 Pains burn and sting, with
puffy swelling. Worse for heat of any
kind.

Lachesis 6 or 30 Excessive pain, much
worse for touch of clothes. Skin looks
blue.

Externally: **Hypercal mother tincture.**
Use as described above.

Gangrene

*The affected part begins to decay and
eventually dies through loss of blood
supply. Can be caused by injuries or
frostbite or occur with certain diseases
such as diabetes. (See also Frostbite).*

Remedies

Arsenicum 30 or 200 Decaying skin
looks black and has an extremely
offensive, putrid smell. The
person is often very restless
and anxious.

Carbo Veg 30 or 200 Useful
remedy for older people who
don't properly recover from
an illness or surgery. May
begin in fingers and toes.
Affected parts are blue with
burning pains and, although they are
cold externally, fanning with cool air
relieves them.

Echinacea 6 Foul-smelling discharge
from the part. Muscular weakness with
aching, tiredness and slowness.
Echinacea is a powerful blood cleanser
and natural antibiotic and can be
taken, either in tincture form or low
potency, in conjunction with other
remedies. It can also be used externally
in tincture form as an antiseptic wash.

Lachesis 30 or 200 Great sensitivity to
touch. Parts look mottled or bluish-
purple. Diabetic ulcers turn
gangrenous. Symptoms are often worse
on falling to sleep or on waking.

Hypercal mother tincture
Dilute 5–10 drops to 300
ml/½ pint/1¼ cups water
and bathe the area.

Hypercal ointment can
be liberally applied
afterwards.

German Measles
(Rubella)

*This is a mild viral infectious illness
which normally begins with a runny
nose, headache and slight fever, and
swollen lymph glands in the neck and
behind the ears. A rash of small red
spots is usually seen first on the face,
neck and chest, then spreads over the
whole body. The incubation period is
two to three weeks and it is contagious
for about one week before and four
days after the onset of the rash.
Although uncomplicated in children, it
is a potential danger if a woman
develops rubella in the first three
months of pregnancy, as it may give
rise to congenital defects such as
deafness, blindness and cleft palate. It
is far better for a girl to contract the
disease in childhood, as this usually
gives life-long immunity; in adulthood
a blood test will show if there is
natural immunity. The vaccine can
damage the foetus if taken during the
first three months of pregnancy.*

Remedies

Aconite 6 or 30 *See* Fevers.
Belladonna 6 or 30 *See* Fevers.
Pulsatilla 6 or 30 Weepy child who
wants company and cuddles. Feels
better outdoors. Usually thirstless.

Gout

*This is an accumulation of uric
acid, usually around the joint of the
big toe, although other small joints
may also be affected. There is
inflammation and extreme pain.
Attention to diet can be very
beneficial, as over-indulgence in
alcohol, tobacco and meat
are known to be triggers.
Constitutional
homeopathic
treatment is
recommended.*

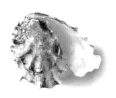
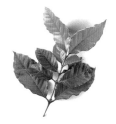

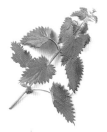
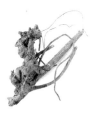

Remedies

Nat Phos 6x and Nat Sulph 6x
Both of these help in the elimination of acid deposits in the body and can be taken in alternation.

Haemorrhage

*Remedies can do much to reduce the loss of blood from a wound, but **seek professional help urgently in serious situations.** If an arm or leg is damaged, prop the limb up to prevent unnecessary loss of blood. Apply firm pressure over the wound. (See also Accidents and Emergencies, Dentist, Nosebleeds.)*

Remedies

Arnica 6 or 30 Bleeding after an injury. Also helps with shock.
China 6 Weakness and exhaustion from loss of blood.
Carbo Veg 6 or 30 Sudden collapse. Person is cold, with cold, clammy sweat, and has a desire for air and to be fanned. Blood is dark.
Ipecac 6 or 30 Loss of bright red blood, with nausea.
Phosphorus 6 or 30 Small wounds bleed more than you would expect. Nosebleeds instead of menses.
Externally: **Ferrum Phos 6x** For small wounds such as a cut finger, crush a few pills and sprinkle over the area, or apply **Calendula mother tincture** neat on cotton wool. These can prevent blood loss from small wounds.

Haemorrhoids (Piles)

Haemorrhoids, or piles, are veins in the rectal area which have become stretched and lost their elasticity. They may protrude, bleed, itch and can sometimes cause excruciating pain. They can be brought on by compression of the veins in the pelvis during pregnancy, aggravated by bowel movements which then, because of fear of pain, lead to constipation, or they may be a symptom of a more serious underlying condition.

Remedies

Aesculus 6 or 30 Piles look like a bunch of purple grapes. Rectum burns and feels full of small sticks. Bleeding piles with sharp shooting pains up the back.
Arnica 6 or 30 Piles after childbirth.
Nit Ac 6 or 30 Easily bleeding piles with tearing pain, or sticking like splinters or needles. Cutting pain after stools.
Nux Vomica 6 or 30 Blind piles which itch and are relieved by cool bathing. Irritable, constipated person, with unsatisfactory urging to pass a stool. Sedentary lifestyle.
Sulphur 6 or 30 Burning, itching and rawness which become worse at night with the warmth of the bed, and by standing or having a bath. Redness around the anus.
Externally: **Aesculus** and **Hamamelis ointment.**
Calendula mother tincture or **Hamamelis mother tincture** to bathe anal area.

Hangovers

The typical symptoms of a hangover (nausea, headache, dizziness, thirst, dry mouth, irritability) are the liver's way of complaining that it is overloaded with toxins. The following remedies may give some relief, but if hangovers occur regularly, try addressing the maintaining cause, which can be helped with constitutional prescribing.

Remedies

Cocculus 6 or 30 Nausea with dizziness and drowsiness.
Nat Phos 6x This tissue salt helps neutralize acidity in the body.
Nat Sulph 6x Cleanses the liver by helping to remove toxins.
Nux Vomica 6 or 30 Bad-tempered. Irritated by light, noise and smells.

Hay Fever

An allergic condition affecting the mucous membranes of the eyes, nose and air passages in people who are over-sensitive to pollens and grasses. Inherited factors play a part; therefore treatment to deal with underlying causes is recommended. Typical symptoms are a runny nose or eyes with a stuffed-up sensation, and itching of eyes, nose or throat.

Remedies

Allium Cepa 6 Frequent sneezing with heavy, burning nasal discharge. Bland, watery secretions from the eyes. The smell of flowers aggravates.
Euphrasia 6 Red, burning, itching, watering eyes. Discharges have the reverse effect of Allium Cepa – water from the eyes burns the skin, but the nasal discharge is

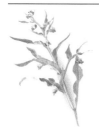
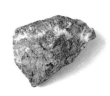
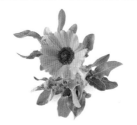
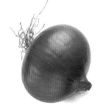
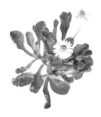

bland. Worse in sunlight and warmth. Better in the open air.

Externally: **Euphrasia mother tincture** Dilute 2 drops in an eyebath and bathe eyes.

Headaches

Headaches may be a warning that something needs to be changed in the person's lifestyle. Missing meals, stress from overworking or worrying are major factors. Over-eating, or indulging in rich, fatty foods, alcohol, coffee, tea or tobacco, all place a strain on the liver, increasing toxicity in the blood which may then be carried to the head. Other triggers include food additives, drugs and environmental pollutants. Some relief may be found by massaging the neck, shoulders and feet, walking barefoot on grass to discharge negative energy back into the earth, or placing your feet in a bowl of cold water, which helps to draw heat down from your head. (See also Head Injuries, Sunstroke.)

CAUTION: Always seek professional help for long-lasting, persistent headaches.

Remedies

Arnica 6 or 30 Headaches caused by a blow to the head.
Arsenicum 6 Headaches which come on after excitement or at weekends. The person is restless and anxious.

Belladonna 6 Sudden violent throbbing, pounding headache. May be feverish with a red face. Worse from being jarred, particularly going downstairs; better from sitting and drawing head backwards. Eyes extremely sensitive to light. Throbbing in the arteries. Sun headaches.
Bryonia 6 Worse for slightest movement, even of eyes. Bursting, splitting headache. An irritable, thirsty person.
Gelsemium 6 Dull heavy headache begins in neck and may settle like a band around the head. Difficult to hold head up. Brought on by mental stress or apprehension. Headache better from frequent urination.
Nux Vomica 6 Splitting headache with nausea. Useful after overindulgence in rich food or alcohol. Feels better by being warm in bed. Oversensitive, irritable people.
Pulsatilla 6 Headaches when digestive system is overburdened, especially after rich food or ices; or a headache instead of the usual menstruation. Better walking in open air. Often tearful and likes to be comforted.

Head Injuries

*If the person is unconscious, turn on to their side to avoid inhalation of fluid. Move the jaw forwards to prevent the tongue from blocking the throat, and check for false teeth. Give Arnica first as it helps to reabsorb blood clots caused by injury. **Seek immediate professional help.** (See also Accidents and Emergencies, Headaches.)*

Remedies

Arnica 30 or 200 Always the first remedy to give where there has been injury. Deals with shock and any bruising to muscles and connective tissue. Other remedies may also be needed.
Hypericum 6 or 30 Bruising to the nerves of the spinal column. Agonizing pain. Follows on after Arnica.
Nat Sulph 6 or 30 Mental troubles or headaches which come on after injury to the head.

Hoarseness and Loss of Voice

Nervousness can sometimes cause complete temporary loss of voice. Coughs and colds can cause inflammation of the larynx (voice box), resulting in hoarseness.

Remedies

Arg Nit 6 or 30 Hoarseness and voice loss from anxiety and apprehension. Worse in a hot, crowded room; craves cool air.
Causticum 6 or 30 Hoarseness worse in the morning, better for talking. Useful for singers or public speakers. Tickling in throat relieved by sipping cold water.
Phosphorus 6 or 30 Hoarseness worse in the evening and on moving from warm to cold air.

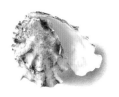
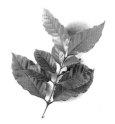

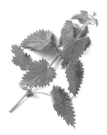
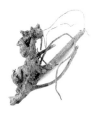

Immunization

There is growing evidence which points to the connection between immunization and long-term chronic diseases. This connection had already been made as far back as the 1870s, when the effects of smallpox vaccination were being documented. At that time homeopaths began to use the term 'vaccinosis' to describe the group of symptoms which came on after vaccination. Many parents know that their children have allergic reactions to immunization: colds, coughs and earaches may develop, with fever or even collapse (anaphylactic shock) which is sometimes fatal. (See relevant sections, including Fever, Shock, Tetanus, Travel, Typhoid.) Children with strong immune systems are better equipped to ward off childhood illness. In homeopathically treated children, the infectious diseases are often experienced in a milder form. Illnesses such as chickenpox or measles are considered by homeopaths to be an opportunity to throw off inherited taints of disease, a bit like having a spring clean.

Incontinence

See *Bedwetting*.

Indigestion

A variety of symptoms can be triggered by careless eating habits, heavy smoking or drugs, or when experiencing emotional upsets such as anger, sadness or anxiety. These include heartburn, acidity, flatulence, nausea and pain. Seek professional advice if any of these become longstanding as they may be masking a more serious complaint.

Remedies

Bryonia 6 Dry tongue, bitter risings and bitter taste in mouth. There is a weight like a stone in the stomach. Although thirsty, cold water may be vomited as soon as it is drunk. Warm drinks and the slightest movement disagree.

Carbo Veg 6 Constant flatulence and heartburn after eating rich or fatty foods, and meat. Slow digestion. Everything turns to gas. Rancid, sour taste on belching, which gives relief. Burning in stomach, extends to back. Bloated abdomen, which feels worse on lying down at night.

China 6 Constant belching with no relief (unlike Carbo Veg). Bitter or sour eructations. Feels full up all the time. Fruit, milk and tea disagree. Relief from bending double.

Kali Mur 6x Indigestion from fats or rich food, with heaviness in stomach. White tongue.

Lycopodium 6 Any food made from flour disagrees. Burning in throat lasts for hours. Fullness after eating very little, which leads to rumbling and release of gas downwards. The Lycopodium person likes very hot food and drinks.

Nat Phos 6x Sour risings and acidity. Yellow, creamy tongue. Worse for eating sugary foods, fat and milk.

Nux Vomica 6 Hiccoughs and indigestion from overindulgence of coffee, alcohol and rich food. Heaviness in stomach and chest a couple of hours after eating. A bitter, sour taste in mouth. A liverish, irritable person.

Pulsatilla 6 Weight like a stone in stomach. Rich, fatty food disagree. Bad taste in the morning. Craves acids and refreshing things. Thirstless.

Infection

See *Abscesses, Blood Poisoning*.

Injuries

See *Accidents and Emergencies*.

Insect Bites

See *Bites and Stings*.

Insomnia

See *Sleep*.

Irritability

This is often a sign of an overworked person with an out-of-balance liver, or hormonal imbalance within the menstrual cycle. Remedies suggested here are for short-term use; any long-standing mental or emotional disequilibrium can best be helped by regular visits to a homeopath, where the whole background can be considered.

Remedies

Bryonia 6 or 30 An irritable person who prefers to be left alone. Worse for any kind of movement, including talking. Dryness anywhere. Feels better on cloudy, damp days.

Kali Carb 6 or 30 Irritability with weakness and backache. Weakness which remains after childbirth or miscarriage.

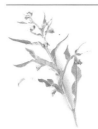 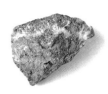 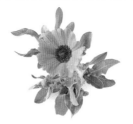 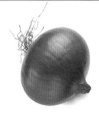 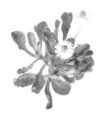

Lycopodium 6 or 30 Awakes angry and irritable. May be domineering at home, although indecisive and lacking in confidence in other areas of life.

Nux Vomica 6 or 30 Angry and impatient. Nagging, faultfinding person. Irritated by noise, light, smells. Headstrong.

Sepia 6 or 30 Snappy and irritable especially before menses. Very easily offended. Wants to be left alone. Sags physically and mentally; overburdened by demands.

Staphysagria 6 or 30 Extremely sensitive to what others say about them. Offended very easily and feel deep indignation. Complaints which come on when anger is unexpressed.

Jetlag and Jet Travel

Jetlag occurs when a person travels rapidly around the globe and becomes out of sync with their body clock. This results in a 'spaced out' state of mind. Sleep is often all that is needed to 'reset' the body clock, but if time is in short supply, Arnica will help to focus awareness back into the immediate surroundings.

Remedies

Arnica 30 For when you feel your body has arrived but *you* haven't. Take 1 tablet 2 times daily for 2 days before your journey; 1 tablet 3 times daily on the day of travel, and 2 times daily for a further 2 days after arrival.

Kali Mur 6x This helps prevent ear pain caused by being at high altitude. Take 1 tablet 2 hours before your flight and another when you first get on the plane. Repeat as necessary.

Kali Phos 6x For tension and difficulty sleeping after your journey. Kali Phos soothes the nervous system. Take 1 every 4 hours on the first day, then 3 times daily for a few days.

Nat Mur 6x Nat Mur helps with water distribution in the body. Take it for swollen ankles or puffy fingers; 1 dose 2 times daily for 2 days before and 2 days after, and 4 times on your day of travel.

Joints

Acute episodes of pain in the joints with disorders such as rheumatism and arthritis can be considerably alleviated with homeopathic remedies, but for lasting benefit the deep-seated causes need to be addressed with constitutional treatment.

Remedies

Aconite 6 or 30 Shooting, tearing pain in the joints which comes on suddenly in very cold, dry weather. Person may be very anxious and restless.

Arnica 6 or 30 Rheumatic pain which comes after injury or over-straining. Sore, bruised pains.

Belladonna 6 or 30 Acute inflammatory rheumatism. Joints are hot, red and sore, and burn. Pains come and go suddenly. May be worse after getting head wet. Motion and jarring aggravate.

Bryonia 6 or 30 Stiffness and stitching pains, with swelling and heat in the joints. Worse from the slightest movement. Irritable and prefers to be left alone.

Causticum 6 or 30 Burning pain which comes on in cold, dry weather and feels better in wet weather (unusual). Rheumatism in the jaw bones.

Ferrum Phos 6x Relieves local congestion, inflammation and throbbing pain.

Nat Phos 6x Neutralizes acid deposits. Use in alternation with Nat Sulph; one dose of each 3 times daily for 10 days.

Nat Sulph 6x Helps the removal of normal waste products in body fluids, accumulation of which causes auto-intoxication.

Rhus Tox 6 or 30 Exposure to cold, wet weather brings on stiff, hot swollen joints. Pains are tearing, shooting, stitching, and worse at night. Gets stiff from sitting too long. The only relief is from warmth and constant movement, even though initial movement aggravates.

Labour

The onset of labour can be a shock or cause fear or excitement, especially if it is the woman's first birth, or begins earlier than anticipated. Progress may be very slow with little dilation of the cervix, or it may be extremely fast, leading to exhaustion. Select a few remedies from those suggested here or buy a Birthing Kit (see page 13).

Remedies

Aconite 6 or 30 For shock and fear with restlessness and anguish. May even say she fears she will die.

Arnica 30 or 200 Shock, bruising and haemorrhage are its three main spheres

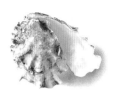
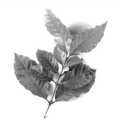

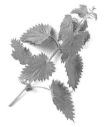
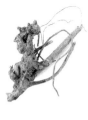

of action in labour. Take one at the beginning of labour and it will help prepare the body for the effort it is about to go through. Soreness and bruising, and any tendency to haemorrhage, will be reduced. Take another 2 or 3 doses of Arnica after the delivery and continue for a further 2 or 3 days (or Bellis Perennis if Arnica doesn't seem to be helping – *see* Surgery).

Carbo Veg 6 or 30 Exhaustion during or after a long delivery. Great desire for moving air (or to be fanned).

Caulophyllum 30 or 200 Very slow or little progress. Weak, irregular contractions. Muscular weakness with trembling or nervous excitement after long, exhausting labour. Useful when womb does not contract immediately after birth (atony).

Causticum 6 or 30 After an episiotomy – the wound is raw and sore and feels like a burn. There may be temporary paralysis of the bladder after labour or surgery, causing retention of urine or incontinence on coughing or sneezing.

Chamomilla 30 or 200 Abrupt and abusive, doesn't want to be touched. Pain is intolerable, unbearable. Very hard to please. Sends everyone out of the room, and then calls them back.

Cimicifuga 30 or 200 Pains dart about, side to side, or down from hips to thighs. A sense of gloom and pessimism. 'I can't do it.' Fear that something terrible will happen. Talkative, fidgety, excitable.

Gelsemium 30 or 200 Uterus feels heavy and sore. Pains extend to the back and hips. Similar to Caulophyllum, with muscular exhaustion and nervous excitement, as in stage fright. There is trembling, and

teeth chatter. May be helpful where the baby is in a posterior positon.

Nat Mur 30 or 200 Prefers to be on her own and may ask everyone to leave the room. Emotionally closed, with a tendency to hold on to past hurts. A negative outlook.

Nux Vomica 30 or 200 Irritated by draughts, noise, smells and light. Doesn't want the windows open (unusual in labour). May feel pressure to empty bowels with each contraction. Tendency to find fault.

Pulsatilla 30 or 200 A tearful person who may invite several friends to the birth. Changeable moods reflected in pains, which fly here and there. Troubled by being in a hot room; wants fresh air.

Externally: **Calendula** (or **Hypercal**) **mother tincture** Soak a sponge in a hot solution of Calendula and bathe the perineum throughout labour; this is very soothing and helps prevent infection after a forceps delivery.

Lumbago

See *Backache*.

Mastitis

See *Breastfeeding*.

Measles

Measles is spread by droplet infection. It incubates for 10–12 days, and is infectious from 2–4 days before the rash appears, and up to 5 days afterwards. Fever, watering inflamed eyes, runny nose, sore throat and sneezing may all be present at the beginning. Then the rash develops on the face and behind the ears and neck, and spreads to the body and limbs. Sometimes small white spots can be seen inside the cheeks. Secondary infections can lead to earache, pneumonia and brain inflammation.

Remedies

Aconite 6 or 30 Useful at the beginning when you are not sure it's measles. There is restlessness with fever, dry croupy or barking cough, redness of the eyes, nasal discharge, which have all appeared suddenly.

Belladonna 6 or 30 Bright red rash, skin burning hot and dry. May be delerious, with throbbing headache.

Bryonia 6 or 30 Rash appears late or disappears too soon. A dry, painful cough. Bronchitis or pneumonia may develop. Children may scream if they are moved because all movement hurts.

Euphrasia 6 or 30 This remedy affects the mucous membranes, particularly the eyes, which stream with burning tears; there is sensitivity to light and a runny nose.

Gelsemium 6 or 30 Gradual onset of fever and chilliness. No desire to move because of exhaustion. Heaviness and aching everywhere. Looks drowsy, with heavy eyelids and a dusky red face. Thirstless but may urinate frequently.

Pulsatilla 6 or 30 Catarrhal symptoms prominent with lack of thirst. There is a thick yellow discharge from the eyes. The child is tearful or whines a lot and wants constant attention.

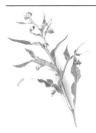
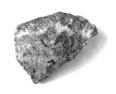
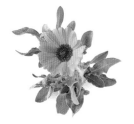
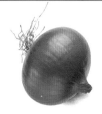
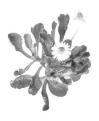

Menstruation

There are many myths linking female problems with the idea of suffering. Consequently some women think it is normal to have painful periods, but when the underlying causes are treated, the pain heals. Remedies given here are suggested for the acute pain.

Remedies

Belladonna 6 or 30 Violent bearing down with cramp and throbbing pain, as if uterus would fall out. Much worse for the slightest jarring, and touch. Feel better standing or sitting erect. Hot gushes of blood. Breasts swollen, hot and tender. Pains come and go suddenly.

Chamomilla 6 or 30 Bad-tempered and very hard to please. Colicky pain before and during the period which may extend down the thighs. Symptoms may come on after being angry. Sufferers 'can't bear it'.

Cocculus 6 or 30 Cramp during and after menses. Weakness, can scarcely stand. Blood gushes out on standing up. Dizziness with nausea. A feeling of emptiness or hollowness in abdomen.

Lachesis 6 or 30 All symptoms are very much better immediately the flow of blood begins. Worse for being in a hot room. Left-sided pain.

Mag Phos 6x or 30 Sudden, sharp, shooting pains and cramps which are relieved with applied heat, gentle pressure and doubling up. Dissolve remedy in warm water and sip.

Nux Vomica 6 or 30 Menstrual cramps may extend all over the body. Constant pressure to empty bowels. Lumbar aches as if back is breaking. Periods are heavy, may be early and

prolonged. Tendency to faint during menses.

Pulsatilla 6 or 30 Pain during and after menses. Pains constantly change location. The person is tearful and feels better for being in company.

Sepia 6 or 30 Snappy and irritable before menses. Better alone.

Migraine

See *Headaches*.

Miscarriage

One of the main causes of a spontaneous abortion, or miscarriage, is a lack of progesterone. Disturbances of the hormonal system can be due to accidents, shock, strong emotional upset or after acute illness. Tests such as amniocentesis or chorionic villus sampling (CVS) to check for chromosomal or genetic disorders may also be factors involved. Always seek professional help if you suddenly begin to bleed and there is also pain present. Consider one of the following remedies for the immediate shock. (See also Abortion.)

Remedies

Aconite 30 or 200 A threatened miscarriage after a shock or fright. The person is extremely anxious and feels she may die.

Arnica 30 or 200 Haemorrhage after an injury or accident, or after sex.

Chamomilla 30 or 200 Miscarriage which is triggered after being angry.

Gelsemium 30 or 200 From fright, excitement or sudden depression. Uterus feels heavy and sore. Nervous chills up and down back. There may be

drowsiness and no thirst.

Pulsatilla 30 or 200 Dark red blood. Changeable symptoms, pains fly here and there. Cannot lie with head low. A tearful person who wants to be comforted. Feels worse in a hot room; wants windows open.

Morning Sickness

The main trigger of nausea and vomiting in pregnancy is hormonal change in the body. It can occur at any time of the day, but is most common in the morning. The eating of dry toast on waking can be helpful. Normally it disappears after the first three months, but if it remains persistent, dehydration and weight loss will affect the growing baby, as well as the mother. It may then be necessary to have fluid replaced intravenously in hospital. The following will help to restore your body fluids. (See also Nausea and Vomiting.)

To 600 ml/1 pint/2½ cups of water add ½ teaspoon salt and ½ teaspoon honey. Every 15 minutes take 1 teaspoon for four doses, followed by 2 teaspoons every 15 minutes for four doses, and finally 3 teaspoons every 15 minutes for four doses.

Remedies

Anacardium 6 or 30 Nausea better from eating. Loss of appetite may alternate with intense emptiness and hunger.

Ant Tart 6 or 30 Waves of nausea, violent retching and vomiting in the morning, better lying on right side. Weakness, exhaustion and drowsiness with all complaints. White mucus may be present. Feels better for vomiting.

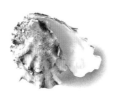
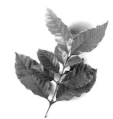
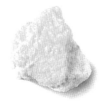
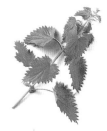
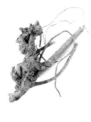

Craves apples and acids.

Ipecac 6 or 30 Excessive salivation with extreme nausea, worse after eating. Vomiting is difficult and doesn't relieve. Lack of thirst. Pork and rich food, fruit, raisins and salad aggravate.

Nat Phos 6x An acid neutralizer. Sour risings with nausea or vomiting. Worse for milk, sugar and fatty foods.

Nux Vomica 6 or 30 Violent retching which is relieved by vomiting; sour, bitter-tasting vomit. Worse in the morning and from noise and smells. Food feels heavy in the stomach, and must loosen clothing. Irritable, constipated person.

Petroleum 6 or 30 Nausea, worse in open air.

Pulsatilla 6 or 30 Nausea and vomiting which comes on in the evening. Food lies like a stone in stomach. Aversion to water, fats, pork, warm food and drink. Prefers to be outdoors in cool air.

Sepia 6 or 30 Nausea at the thought or smell of food, worse in the morning, or from rinsing the mouth. Craving for vinegar, pickles. Symptoms are not relieved by eating. May feel mentally and physically dragged down.

Mouth Ulcers

Also called canker sores. Found on the tongue, gums or inner cheeks, they can be very painful, and may indicate a run-down state of health or poor diet. Frequent occurrence can be helped with regular constitutional treatment.

Remedies

Kali Mur 6x White ulcers, with a white-coated tongue.

Merc Sol 6 or 30 There may be a metallic taste, extra saliva and offensive breath with mouth ulcers. The tongue is often broad and flabby.

Nat Mur 6x Blisters and ulcers which smart and burn in mouth and on tongue.

Mumps

Mumps is a viral infection which has an incubation period of two or three weeks. It begins with flu-like symptoms, mild fever and sore throat. Swelling appears in the glands just below and in front of the earlobes. It is infectious for two or three days before the glands swell and until the swelling has gone. Symptoms are usually mild and short-lasting, but it may spread to breasts, ovaries or testicles, and sometimes causes sterility in men.

Remedies

Aconite 6 or 30 Useful at the beginning where there is sudden onset of fever, with restlessness and a big thirst.

Belladonna 6 or 30 Thirsty for lemonade. Dry burning heat, bright red face. Swelling more on the right side, with violent shooting pains. Delirium may be present, with sensitivity to light.

Carbo Veg 6 or 30 Where there is involvement of breasts, ovaries or testicles. Person is chilly but wants plenty of moving air.

Merc Sol 6 or 30 Offensive sweat and breath, foul taste in mouth, often with increased saliva.

Phytolacca 6 or 30 Pain shoots into the ear on swallowing. Face looks pale. Glands feel stony hard.

Pulsatilla 6 or 30 Mumps which spreads to the breasts, ovaries or testicles. The person craves fresh air; children are tearful or whine a lot and become clingy. Worse in a warm room.

Rhus Tox 6 or 30 Mumps on the left side. Worse at night and when resting. May come on in cold wet weather. There are cold sores on the lips.

Nails

Silica is a constituent of nails and if taken in homeopathic dilution can help to strengthen them. Take 1 Silica 6× 2 times daily for 2 weeks. This can be repeated infrequently.
SEE CAUTION regarding use of Silica (page 81).

Nausea and Vomiting

*Nausea is the sensation of feeling sick or being about to vomit. Vomiting is a reflex action when abdominal muscles contract, causing the stomach to eject its contents. Causes for either of these conditions range from minor things such as eating rich or contaminated food to serious stomach disease, and can also be of psychological origin, e.g. from excitement or anxiety. **Repeated vomiting needs professional help** as there may be an intestinal obstruction. Excessive vomiting can quickly lead to loss of salt and water, especially in babies and young children. (See also Morning Sickness.)*

Remedies

Aethusa 6 or 30 Violent, sudden vomiting, especially in pregnancy.

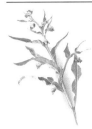
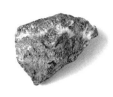
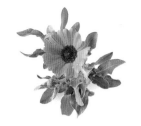
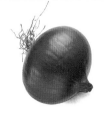
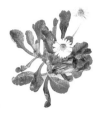

Projectile vomiting of babies from intolerance of milk. They are too weak to hold their heads up, become limp and fall into a deep sleep after vomiting. Can develop during teething.

Arsenicum 6 or 30 Vomiting and diarrhoea caused by food poisoning. Anxious and restless, with burning pains relieved by warm drinks.

Bryonia 6 or 30 Bitter vomiting immediately after eating or drinking. Nausea and vomiting made worse by the slightest movement.

Ipecac 6 or 30 Continuous nausea not relieved by vomiting. The tongue is clean or bright red. Worse from overeating rich food or pork, salads or berries.

Nux Vomica 6 or 30 Nausea which would be relieved from vomiting, if only they could. From over-indulging in food, alcohol, drugs, coffee.

Phosphorus 6 or 30 Vomits as soon as food or drink warms up in the stomach. Ice-cold drinks help pain in the stomach, or vomits from the sight of water.

Pulsatilla 6 or 30 Stomach feels heavy. Worse from rich, fatty food. Vomits food eaten much earlier. No thirst.

Veratrum Alb 6 or 30 Excessive purging from stomach and bowels with cold sweat on forehead. Craves ice-water which is vomited immediately. Of great use in cholera epidemics.

Nervousness

See *Fear and Anxiety.*

Nettle Rash (Urticaria)

An eruption of raised red or white lumpy patches on the skin, with itching which looks as if the person has been stung by nettles. This is sometimes caused by an allergic reaction to certain foods, chemicals, pollutants or an insect sting (see Bites and Stings). By treating the underlying causes, homeopathy can bring changes to the level of susceptibility.

Remedies

Apis 6 or 30 Swellings burn, itch and sting and may come on during fever. Heat aggravates and cold brings relief. Can be used in emergency situations where there is a severe allergic reaction (*see Bites and Stings*).

Rhus Tox 6 or 30 Blistery eruptions which burn, itch and sting, with feverish conditions and joint pains. From getting chilled in wet weather. Cold aggravates, heat relieves.

Urtica Urens 6 or 30 Nettle rash, or prickly heat which is worse every year in the same season. Also caused by bee stings, eating shellfish, and from getting overheated during exercise.

Neuralgia

Neuralgia is a severe shooting pain which originates in a nerve. The most common areas affected are the face, when the trigeminal nerve is involved; and the back and thigh when the sciatic nerve is affected. (See also Backache, Pregnancy – Walking Difficulties.)

Remedies

Ferrum Phos 6x Pain and inflammation at the beginning of feverish illness brought on by getting chilled.

Hypericum 6 or 30 Violent shooting pains, with tingling, burning and numbness. Much worse from touch or change of weather. May be caused by injury.

Kali Phos 6x Acts like a nutrient to the nerves, helps people who are nervy types, and supplements the action of Mag Phos.

Mag Phos 6x An anti-spasmodic remedy. Shooting, darting pain which is relieved by warmth, a hot bath and rubbing. Alternate with Kali Phos until relief is obtained.

Spigelia 6 or 30 Trigeminal neuralgia with violent pains which burn like hot needles and radiate outwards. The pain severely affects the eyes.

Nosebleeds

Causes include injury, fever and high blood pressure. (See also Haemorrhage.)

Remedies

Aconite 6 or 30 Nosebleed of bright red blood, after fright or shock. The nose feels numb.

Arnica 6 or 30 After injury, washing the face or coughing.

Ferrum Phos 6x Bright red blood. Comes on during a headache, fever or coughing.

Hamamelis 6 or 30 Nosebleed of dark blood during fever, or instead of menses.

Nux Vomica 6 or 30 Nosebleed during sleep, from coughing or stooping, and after piles have been removed.

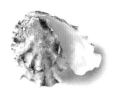
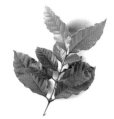

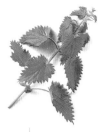
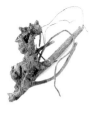

Phosphorus 6 or 30 Person bleeds easily. Nosebleed of bright red blood instead of menstrual period, or when emptying bowels, or during cough.

Pulsatilla 6 or 30 Nosebleed of dark blood. Comes on in a warm room, or after getting wet, and before or during a menstrual period. Nosebleed instead of menses.

Operations

See *Surgery*.

Pain

*The normal reaction to pain is to get rid of it as quickly as possible. However, except in the case of injury or surgery where it is obvious how the pain resulted, we need to look at the underlying cause. Analgesics will only mask the message the pain is trying to give us. **Seek professional help if there is persistent unexplained pain.** (See also Accidents and Emergencies, Backache, Dentist, Headache, Labour, Menstruation, Pregnancy, Neuralgia, Surgery.)*

Remedies

Aconite 6, 30 or 200 Frantic; screams with pain which is intolerable and frightening. Pains come on suddenly, and are burning, tearing with numbness and tingling. Worse for touch and at night, just around midnight. Fear of death.

Arnica 6, 30 or 200 Sore bruised pain. Causes are injuries, over-exertion, shock. Fear of being touched. Denies anything is wrong, even with

serious symptoms.

Chamomilla 6, 30 or 200 Angry, over-sensitive. Can't bear the pain. Demands instant relief. Worse from being looked at.

Coffea 6, 30 or 200 Over-excitable. Cannot bear any pain. Over-sensitive to noise, touch, smells. Wakes at the slightest sound.

Ferrum Phos 6x Throbbing pain which comes on when inflammation is present.

Hepar Sulph 6, 30 or 200 Oversensitive to pain, touch, a cold draught. Slight pain causes fainting. Pains are sore and sharp like splinters. Touchy mentally and physically.

Hypericum 6, 30 or 200 Pains which shoot along nerve pathways after injuries to fingers and toes, or other areas rich in nerves.

Mag Phos 6x, 30 or 200 Paroxysmal pain which shoots like lightning, or cramp which doubles the person up. Relieved by having a hot bath, from pressure and rubbing. This remedy is better dissolved in warm water and sipped.

Palpitations

*Increased awareness of the heart's action, coupled with a faster beat, is common during moments of excitement, anxiety or shock. Tea, coffee, alcohol and tobacco can have the same effect. **If there is no apparent cause, there may be organic heart***

disease; seek professional advice. (See also Fear and Anxiety.)

Remedies

Aconite 6 or 30 Palpitations with great fear and restlessness, after a shock or from getting chilled in cold winds.

Coffea 6 or 30 From extreme excitement, which prevents sleep.

Kali Phos 6x From excitement or worry. Worse from going up stairs.

Nux Vomica 6 or 30 Brought on from drinking coffee.

Panic

See *Fear and Anxiety*.

Period Pains and Cramps

See *Menstruation*.

Piles

See *Haemorrhoids*.

Pre-Menstrual Tension

See *Irritability, Tearfulness*.

Pregnancy

Many disorders of pregnancy can be improved with homeopathic remedies. Regular treatment from a homeopath throughout pregnancy, or by both parents before conception, can help to offset possible future complications in the labour and improve the health of the unborn baby.

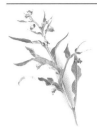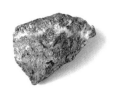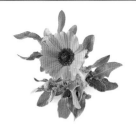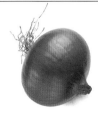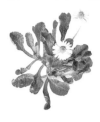

(See also *Backache, Constipation, Haemorrhoids, Indigestion, Labour, Morning Sickness, Nausea and Vomiting, Sleep, Varicose Veins.*) *The following remedies can all be taken at intervals throughout pregnancy. Take 1 tablet 2 times daily for 10 days. Repeat every 1–2 months.*

Remedies

Calc Fluor 6x Extra stretch is what's needed during labour and this remedy will tighten up flabby tissues. Also helps to prevent stretch marks and varicose veins.

Calc Phos 6x Needed for the production of new blood cells, and the nutrition of bones and teeth.

Ferrum Phos 6x and Kali Sulph 6x Both work as oxygen carriers in the blood so are beneficial where there is a tendency towards anaemia. Alternate them, one in the morning and one in the evening.

Nat Mur 6x Thin, watery blood with weakness. Emotionally negative and depressed. May crave salt.

Walking Difficulties in Pregnancy

As the baby grows and ligaments supporting the joints around the uterus soften, there may be pressure on nerves. This can cause backache and severe sharp pain which shoots down the legs. It usually passes quickly, but while it is happening there may be a temporary inability to walk.

Remedies

Bellis Perennis 6 or 30 This is the first remedy to try in this situation, as it has an affinity with abdominal joints, muscles and nerves. Pelvic region feels intensely sore and bruised.

Arnica 6 or 30 Helpful where you feel sore and bruised from the baby's kicking. If Arnica does not relieve, take Bellis Perennis.

Aesculus 6 or 30 Back gives out when walking. Constant backache of sacrum and hips, worse stooping or rising from sitting. Especially where piles are present, indicating congestion in the veins.

Staphysagria 6 or 30 If the baby kicks in such a way that you feel a little indignant about it.

Puncture Wounds

Splinters and accidents from stepping on pins, rusty nails, barbed wire or tools can be dealt with very effectively. (See also Accidents and Emergencies, Bites and Stings, Cuts and Abrasions, Shock and Collapse, Tetanus.)

Remedies

Arnica 6 or 30 Can help bring splinters to the surface and deal with possible shock.

Hepar Sulph 6 or 30 Helps the removal of foreign objects. Wounds turn septic, discharging much foul-smelling pus. Splinter-like pains.

Hypericum 6 or 30 Intense pain shoots up from injured parts which are rich in nerves. If given immediately, can prevent tetanus from developing, but seek professional advice.

Ledum 6 or 30 This remedy also prevents tetanus and can be used for the same injuries as Hypericum, but the part feels cold and is relieved by cold; there is puffiness and a pale, mottled appearance.

Silica 6 or 30 For an obstinate splinter, Silica will help it come to the surface.

Externally: **Calendula** (or **Hypercal**) **mother tincture** Dilute 5–10 drops in 120 ml/4 fl oz/½ cup of water. This will help prevent sepsis from forming.

Rheumatism

See *Backache, Joints.*

Rubella

See *German Measles.*

Sadness

The many causes of sadness and depression all come within the domain of homeopathy. Remedies can help where there is homesickness, loss of a relative or friend from death, loss of work or a pet. Regular constitutional treatment is recommended where the situation is deep-seated. (See also Tearfulness).

Remedies

Ignatia 30 Sadness after bereavement. Brooding, silent grief or becomes hysterical. Laughs at serious things. Sighs a lot.

Nat Mur 30 Depressed and gloomy. Suffers in silence and usually only cries when alone. Gets stuck in past resentments.

Pulsatilla 30 Easy flowing tears, feels much better for company. Easily offended. Changeable moods – crying one minute, laughing the next. Fear when alone. Feels better when walking in the open air.

Scarlet Fever

Scarlet fever, although not commonly

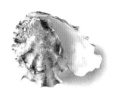
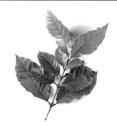

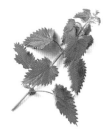
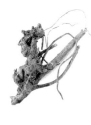

seen nowadays, does still occur. It is an acute infectious disease of childhood with symptoms of high fever, sore, swollen throat, enlarged glands under the jaw, a 'strawberry' tongue and a red rash. There may also be shivering, vomiting and headache, with delerium. The face is flushed, with the area around the mouth remaining pale. The rash of tiny red spots, which merge together to give a scarlet appearance, spreads all over the body. Incubation is usually 2–4 days. There is often a peeling of the skin as other symptoms subside.

Remedies

Belladonna 6 or 30 The main remedy used in the past during epidemics of scarlet fever. Bright red, hot face, red eyes, dilated pupils. Dry, burning heat. Strawberry tongue. Throbbing headache. Belladonna wants to be warm and is thirsty.

Apis 6 or 30 Drowsy, with a sore, swollen, oedematous throat which stings, and is better from cold drinks. Feels worse in a hot room and is usually thirstless.

Rhus Tox 6 or 30 A coarse rash which may develop little blisters. Very restless and sleepy. Worse at night. Better from being warm.

Sciatica

See *Backache and Back Injuries, Neuralgia, Pregnancy – Walking Difficulties.*

Septic Conditions

See *Abscesses, Blood Poisoning.*

Shingles (Herpes Zoster)

This is caused by a similar virus to the one found in chickenpox. Initially, the person feels unwell for a few days, with a slight rise in temperature. Then the eruption of a blistery rash appears along the site of a single nerve, which accounts for the rash being confined to one side of the body. Pain can remain long afterwards.

Remedies

Apis 6 or 30 Large vesicles (blisters) which burn and sting like hot needles. There is a puffy, rosy red appearance to the area. Better for cold applications, worse for warmth and touch. Person is very restless.

Arsenicum 6 or 30 Intense burning pain, relieved by warmth. A fussy, irritable person who feels the cold.

Mezereum 6 or 30 Violent burning and itching; pain which remains after the rash has gone. Much worse at night, from getting warm in bed and from touch.

Rhus Tox 6 or 30 May come on after being out in cold, wet weather. Worse at night, cannot lie still in bed. May feel very despondent.

Staphysagria 6 or 30 Stinging, smarting pain that precedes shingles. Itching changes place on scratching. Much worse from touch. Mentally also very touchy. Symptoms worse when angry.

Shock and Collapse

*If blood pressure falls too low to maintain an adequate flow of blood through the tissues, vital functions begin to close down and this leads to shock. Serious injuries, surgery, allergic reactions, hearing bad news can all cause shock. The most urgent need is to re-oxygenate the brain; do this by placing the person on his or her back with legs slightly raised so that blood drains towards the head, and loosen any tight clothing. **Do not attempt to move a seriously injured person as additional pain will add to the shock.** Symptoms of shock include collapse, confusion, cold pale skin, shallow irregular breathing, and rapid weak pulse. (See also Accidents and Emergencies, Bites and Stings.)*

Remedies

Aconite 6, 30 or 200 Severe shock with great fear and restlessness. Fear is so great, person may scream, or say they will die. Sudden collapse. Useful after surgical shock.

Arnica 6, 30 or 200 Will help the person to regain consciousness, reduces haemorrhage and shock. Give before and after any surgery.

Ignatia 6, 30 or 200 Shock after bad news. May become hysterical.

Rescue Remedy Place a few drops inside the lips, behind the ears or on the wrists.

Sinuses

See *Catarrh and Sinusitis.*

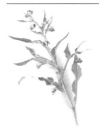
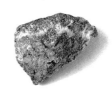
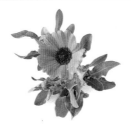
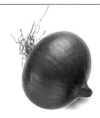
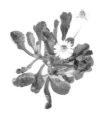

Skin

The skin is an outlet for some of the body's waste products, just as the nose is when we have a cold, or the mouth when we have a cough. From a holistic viewpoint, spots, boils and rashes are an expression of a disorder on another level. Ultimately their purpose is to help us maintain a healthier condition inside. If exit points like the skin are sealed off – for example, when strong medicated ointments are used for disorders such as eczema – toxicity can build up, perhaps leading to more serious illness later in life. Constitutional treatment is recommended. (See also Abscesses, Acne, Athlete's Foot, Bites and Stings, Blood Poisoning, Cold Sores, Nettle Rash, Shingles, Thrush.)

Sleep

If you have difficulty relaxing at bedtime because your mind is over-active, it may help to write a list of your thoughts before getting into bed, or imagine that you are putting them in a container which you place outside the room, knowing that you can return to it in the morning. Then picture your favourite place in nature and imagine you are relaxing there.

Remedies

Arsenicum 6 or 30 Sleepless from anxiety and fear. Tosses and turns, wakes up between midnight and 2 a.m.

Coffea 6 or 30 Sleepless from excitement. All senses more acute. Wakes up from the slightest sound.

Gelsemium 6 or 30 A sense of anticipation about a forthcoming event, such as visiting the dentist, taking a driving test or examination, or the shock of unpleasant news prevents sleep. Frequent desire to empty bladder.

Kali Phos 6x Soothes the nervous system. Take hourly for a few doses before bedtime.

Nux Vomica 6 or 30 An over-active mind prevents sleep, or the person wakes too early and is unable to sleep again.

Sulphur 6 or 30 Difficulty in going to bed early; likes to have catnaps during the day. Wakes unrefreshed and does not want to get up.

Spine

See *Backache.*

Splinters

See *Puncture Wounds.*

Sprains and Strains

If the pain of an injury persists and shows no sign of improvement within 24–36 hours of taking the appropriate homeopathic remedy, seek professional help to check for a fracture.

Remedies

Arnica 6 or 30 For the shock. Bruised, sore pains.

Bellis Perennis 6 or 30 Intense soreness of muscles; useful after gardening, and where swellings or lumps remain after injuries. Deeper-acting than Arnica.

Bryonia 6 or 30 Swollen painful joints, worse for slightest movement.

Ledum 6 or 30 Injuries where the swollen part is cold or numb; feels better for cold application.

Rhus Tox 6 or 30 Useful for torn ligaments and tendons, and connective tissue covering muscles. Parts are hot and swollen. Stiffness comes on from sitting. Feels restless.

Ruta 6 or 30 Similar to Rhus Tox – works on torn tendons and ligaments – and also on bone coverings (periosteum).

Symphytum 6 or 30 Useful after Arnica and Ruta, but if you suspect a fracture, do not give until bone is realigned.

Stiff Neck

Neck stiffness may be caused by getting chilled or wet, sitting in a draught, lying with the head in an uncomfortable position, or from overstraining (see Sprains and Strains). Stress of any kind can also cause neck muscles to constrict, leading to a blockage of energy, which may then present itself as pain. As well as homeopathic remedies, gentle massage to the area may be of benefit.

CAUTION: If pain persists and is accompanied by fever, seek professional help.

Remedies

Aconite 6 or 30 Stiffness caused by being in a cold wind, or sitting in a draught.

Bryonia 6 or 30 Neck pain is worse for touch or movement. Irritable, wants to be left alone.

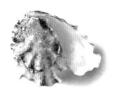 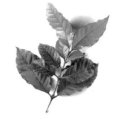 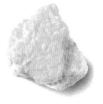 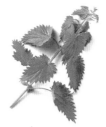 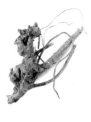

Dulcamara 6 or 30 Worse getting chilled while hot, for example from swimming; sudden changes in weather such as warm days and cold nights in autumn.

Stings

See *Bites*.

Strains

See *Sprains*.

Styes

Styes begin with swelling of the eyelid when there is inflammation around an eyelash. The swelling gradually comes to a head and can discharge pus. The stye may not ripen but instead develop into a hard lump.

Remedies

Apis 6 or 30 Stinging pain which is worse for heat and better for cold applications. The area around the stye may look shiny and swollen.

Hepar Sulph 6 or 30 Sharp pain like a splinter. The person may be irritable and very sensitive to the slightest draught.

Pulsatilla 6 or 30 Styes which have a yellow or green discharge. The person feels worse in a warm room and better in fresh air.

Silica 6 or 30 Styes which are slow to ripen or don't come to a head. May develop into a hard lump.

Staphysagria 6 or 30 Recurrent styes, worse for touch. Particularly useful where there is unexpressed anger.

Externally: **Euphrasia mother tincture**

Relieves soreness and burning of eyes. Dissolve 2 drops in sterile water in an eyebath and bathe eye.

Sunburn

See *Burns*.

Sunstroke

The effects of being over-exposed to the sun can range from mild headaches and tiredness to very serious conditions such as collapse, delirium, or even convulsions. In severe cases, the cooling system of the body becomes traumatized, leading to the dehydration of body tissues and organs, with the possibility of a dangerous rise in body temperature. Other symptoms that indicate sunstroke include dizziness, nausea, vomiting, weakness and rapid pulse rate.

IN SERIOUS CASES: Treat for shock while seeking professional help. Lower the body heat quickly by wrapping person in wet towels or spray with cool water. Use ice packs if available but avoid getting too cold. To help rehydration, drink a cup of water with ½ teaspoon of salt added, or follow details given under Morning Sickness (see page 38).

Remedies

Aconite 30 or 200 For shock, fear and possible convulsions.

Belladonna 30 or 200 Burning heat, redness and dryness. Throbbing

headache with sensitivity to light and noise. Possible convulsions. Better from bending head backwards.

Glonoine 30 or 200 Bursting, pounding headache. Worse from bending head backwards.

Nat Mur 6x Helps with fluid distribution in the body.

Surgery

When homeopathic remedies are used before and immediately after surgery, the healing process is sped up considerably. This can be accompanied by a reduction in post-operative complications such as haemorrhage, inflammation and infection. Bruising to internal organs and deep tissue repairs quickly. Vomiting brought on by anaesthetics may also be prevented. If you are upset after medical intervention, this can be alleviated.

Remedies

Aconite 6 or 30 Great fear and anguish with restlessness. Possible fear of death.

Arnica 30 or 200 Bruised sore pain with fear of being touched (see Bellis Perennis below). Take this remedy immediately before an operation and another dose as soon as possible afterwards.

Bellis Perennis 6 or 30 Bruised, sore pain. This remedy follows on after Arnica where there has been surgery involving deep tissue, e.g. Caesareans.

China 6 Excessive flatulence and bloating; feels no relief from passing gas. Helps intestinal action to return to normal after abdominal operations. Can also be used where there is exhaustion from loss of body fluids.

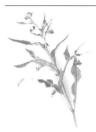
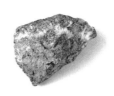
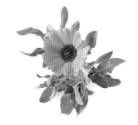
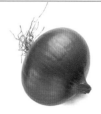
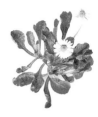

Gelsemium 6 or 30 Anxiety, feeling of dread before an ordeal. Weak and trembly. Heaviness anywhere. Increased urination.

Hypericum 6 or 30 Damage to tissue rich in nerves. Violent pains shoot along nerve pathways.

Phosphorus 6 or 30 Helps prevent post-operative vomiting if taken before operation. Take a second dose after.

Pyrogen 30 or 200 This remedy is invaluable where a severe septic state is developing. Fever with restlessness. Temperature oscillates suddenly. Pains are like those of Arnica – aching, bruised and sore. Person may be confused, imagining they have extra arms and legs.

Staphysagria 6 or 30 Stinging, cutting, smarting pains after surgery. Useful where the person feels as if the body has been invaded or there is a sense of humiliation after a physical examination. Resentment and anger towards hospital staff may be present. *Externally:* **Calendula** (or **Hypercal**) **mother tincture**. The healing of wounds after surgery will be enhanced and sepsis prevented with Calendula. It can be taken internally (6th potency 2 times daily for 5–7 days) and the tincture diluted for bathing the wound. Afterwards Calendula ointment can be gently rubbed in around the edges.

Tearfulness

Tears can act like a safety valve, bringing relief from internal pressures, or be a powerful way of demanding and receiving attention (love). They may stimulate compassion or anger in the bystander. An imbalance of water is shown in people who cry a lot or

who are unable to cry, indicating difficulty with or a damming up of the flow of life.

Remedies

Chamomilla 6 or 30 Cries out from pain or bad temper. Nothing pleases the Chamomilla baby, who wants first one thing, then another.

Ignatia 6 or 30 Oversensitive and highly emotional. Sighing and sobbing, or silent brooding grief after the death of a relative or friend.

Nat Mur 6 or 30 Wants to cry but feels unable to let the tears out. Can cry when alone. Hates fuss.

Pulsatilla 6 or 30 Easily offended, cries at the slightest provocation. Loves sympathy and being cuddled when upset. Worse before menses.

Staphysagria 6 or 30 Sadness without any cause. Always angry. The least word hurts very deeply.

Teething Babies

Some babies (and frequently their parents!) have a painful time during teething, with the babies showing symptoms of fever, coughs, colds, earache, diarrhoea, constipation or skin rashes, coupled with irritability and bad temper. They may refuse food, become clingy and typically have one red, hot cheek, with excessive dribbling. Offer something hard to chew on. Homeopathy can be used to treat both the emotions and the pain.

Remedies

Aethusa 6 or 30 Teething babies who cannot tolerate milk, which is vomited immediately it is swallowed. Hunger follows, or they go limp and fall asleep.

Belladonna 6 or 30 A hot, flushed face; may be feverish and delirious.

Calc Phos 6x Useful if there are no outstanding symptoms to indicate other remedies. Helps the teeth to come through. There may be delayed closure of the fontanelle on the head.

Chamomilla 6 or 30 Pain is unbearable. A very bad-tempered baby. One cheek flushed. Stools turn green.

Ferrum Phos 6x Where there is inflammation, redness and fever.

Merc Sol 6 or 30 Baby is worse at night, with much dribbling. Stools may be slimy and green, with soreness in the nappy area.

Tetanus

*Tetanus is caused by a toxin which can multiply only if there is a lack of oxygen. The **Clostridium tetani** bacillus finds its most suitable environment in the dead tissue of some puncture wounds, such as those caused by rusty nails, barbed wire or while working with the soil or with horses. Symptoms are stiffness in the muscles near the wound, followed by stiffness of the muscles around the jaw, eventually preventing opening of the mouth – known as lockjaw. Bathe the part with Hydrogen Peroxide to oxygenate it. (See also Puncture Wounds.)*

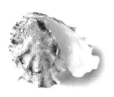 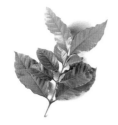  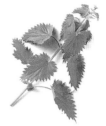 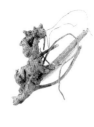

Remedies

Hypericum 30 Pain extends upwards from injured part. If given immediately, Hypericum can prevent tetanus developing. On the first day repeat every 2 hours for 4 doses or until the pain subsides. Take 2 times daily for the following 2–4 days, then if anxious follow instructions for Clostridium Tetani below.

Ledum 30 Coldness of the affected part, which is better for cold. Use in the same way as Hypericum. If you are unsure whether to use Hypericum or Ledum, use both in alternation, as this is a potentially dangerous situation.

Clostridium Tetani 30 Use this as a prophylactic if your travels take you to isolated places. Take 1 dose 2 times weekly for 4 weeks.

Throat

Continually occurring sore throats and tonsillitis respond well to constitutional homeopathic treatment. The following remedies will help some of the acute stages.

Remedies

Aconite 6 or 30 Sudden acute inflammation, after exposure to cold, dry wind. There may be great restlessness and anxiety.

Apis 6 or 30 Stinging pains, with watery-looking swelling in throat. Worse from warm drinks, better from cold. Feels worse in a warm room.

Arsenicum 6 or 30 Burning throat which is relieved with warm drinks. Very chilly person, restless and weak.

Baptisia 6 or 30 The person looks very drowsy, as if drugged. Sore throat accompanied with flu-like symptoms of heavy, aching muscles. Throat is dark red, may be ulcerated.

Belladonna 6 or 30 Heat, redness, congestion and dryness are typical of this remedy. Tonsils are inflamed and bright red. There may be a throbbing headache.

Dulcamara 6 or 30 Every cold settles in the throat or eyes, or affects the bladder. Symptoms come on after sudden changes in the weather, or from being chilled while hot in summer, even from eating ice cream. Throat fills with mucus.

Ferrum Phos 6x For the beginning of inflammation. Burning rawness which is worse on empty swallowing; hoarseness.

Hepar Sulph 6 or 30 Swelling of tonsils and neck glands. Pain as if a fishbone or splinter is sticking in the throat, which extends to the ears on swallowing. Irritable and feels worse from the slightest draught; wraps head warmly.

Kali Mur 6x Greyish-white ulcers in throat, with thick white mucus.

Lachesis 6 or 30 Throat symptoms begin on left and may move to the right. 'Empty' swallowing is much more difficult than swallowing food. Hot drinks are unbearable.

Lycopodium 6 or 30 Right-sided, or extends right to left. Soreness is worse from cold and better from warm drinks. Feels like a lump stuck in throat.

Merc Sol 6 or 30 Ulcerated throat which smarts and burns. Increased saliva, bad breath and discharges. Sweats without relief.

Thrush

*Thrush, or yeast infection, comes about when the healthy bacteria in the mouth, intestines or vagina are reduced, perhaps after a dose of antibiotics. This then allows the fungus **Candida albicans** to multiply. There are characteristic white patches in the mouth, or a thick, often white, curdy discharge, with itching and soreness which passes between sexual partners. Bathing the area with live yoghurt or adding half a cup of vinegar to the bath can be very soothing. Calendula mother tincture also provides relief.*

Remedies

Kali Mur 6x A white tongue, with milky white patches in the mouth.

Kreosotum 6 or 30 A lumpy, gushing, smelly discharge with violent itching and burning of the vulva and vagina.

Nit Ac 6 or 30 Tremendous itching and burning of the vagina after sexual intercourse.

Pulsatilla 6 or 30 Discharge may be watery, yellow-green, or thick like cream, with back pain.

Sepia 6 or 30 Offensive lumpy, yellow-green discharge with weak back and dragging down in the abdomen. An irritable, exhausted person.

Tonsillitis

See *Throat*.

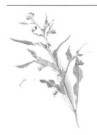
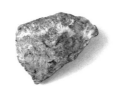
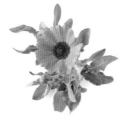
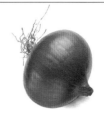
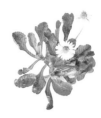

Toothache

Dental decay is not the only cause of tooth pain. Tension, anxiety and anger may also bring it on. While visiting the dentist, remedies can be used instead of antibiotics to heal an abscess and reduce pain. There is a vast number of remedies covering toothache; only a small selection is given here. (See also Abscesses, Dentist, Teething Babies.)

Remedies

Aconite 6 or 30 Toothache which comes after being out in cold, dry winds.

Arnica 6 or 30 Bruised, sore pain after visiting the dentist.

Chamomilla 6 or 30 Pain better from ice-cold water.

Hepar Sulph 6 or 30 Pain from an abscess which discharges foul pus. Worse for taking cold drinks and food, and from the slightest cold draught. Splinter-like pains.

Mag Phos 6x or 30 Relief from heat in any form. Pains shoot like lightning.

Pulsatilla 6 or 30 Pain better for cold water and worse for heat in any form.

Silica 6 or 30 Toothache with swollen face and glands. Abscess at the root of the teeth. Wants face to be warm.

Travel

Although it is possible to buy homeopathic remedies in an increasing number of countries, it is convenient to have your own first-aid kit which suits your specific needs (see page 13). Remedies can also have a prophylactic use and may be used instead of immunization; consult a professional homeopath for advice (and see Immunization). (See also Accidents and Emergencies, Bites and Stings, Blood Poisoning, Diarrhoea, Jetlag and Jet Travel, Nausea and Vomiting, Tetanus, Travel Sickness, Typhoid.)

Travel Sickness

Information is given for alleviating acute symptoms, but lasting benefit will be achieved by having constitutional treatment.

Remedies

Cocculus 6 or 30 Feels faint and dizzy with nausea and vomiting. Worse in the open air, better lying down. A hollow sensation in the head or abdomen.

Petroleum 6 or 30 Dreads the open air. Better lying with head high.

Tabacum 6 or 30 Worse opening eyes. Better in the fresh air.

Typhoid

*Typhoid fever is an infectious condition brought on by the **Salmonella typhi** bacillus. It is carried in contaminated food or drinking water in areas with poor sanitation. The onset of symptoms include headache, lassitude, sleeplessness and fever at night. As the illness develops, there may be blood in the stools from ulceration and perforation of the small intestine, enlargement of the spleen, inflammation of the gall bladder and lungs.*

Remedies

Baptisia 30 One of the main remedies for typhoid fever. There is a general septic state with aching, soreness of muscles. The person deteriorates rapidly. Mucous membranes become dark. Looks drowsy and confused. Falls asleep while speaking. Feels as if parts are separated. Can be used prophylactically – take one dose every week while travelling. It also helps to antidote the bad effects of anti-typhoid serum injections.

Salmonella Typhi 30 Take this instead of Baptisia once weekly while travelling in risky areas.

Urticaria

See *Nettle Rash*.

Vaccination

See *Immunization*.

Varicose veins

The tendency towards varicose veins is often hereditary, and they can be brought on if the person's work requires many hours standing, or in pregnancy where there is pressure by the foetus on internal organs. When blood stagnates in the veins, they become swollen and stretched. They can develop on the testicles (known as variocele), on the vulva and at the lower end of the bowel (piles), as well as on the legs. The underlying causes need constitutional treatment.

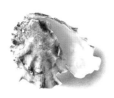
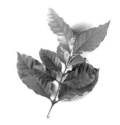
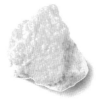
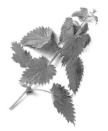
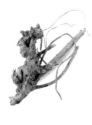

Remedies

Calc Fluor 6x Increases elasticity in the walls of the veins. Take twice daily for 2 weeks. Can be repeated at lengthy intervals.

Hamamelis 6 This remedy's main area of action is the veins, especially of the rectum, genitals and limbs. There is bruised soreness with a bursting sensation. The pain is prickling and stinging, and the part is hard and knotted.

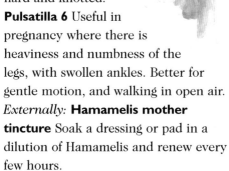

Pulsatilla 6 Useful in pregnancy where there is heaviness and numbness of the legs, with swollen ankles. Better for gentle motion, and walking in open air. *Externally:* **Hamamelis mother tincture** Soak a dressing or pad in a dilution of Hamamelis and renew every few hours.

Vertigo

Caused by a disturbance in the ears when the power of balance is lost. Can be made worse by lack of sleep, or food, or from overworking. Objects appear to move or the person feels that he or she is moving. (See also Travel Sickness.)

Remedies

Borax 6 or 30 Worse going up or down stairs. Babies dislike downward or upward motion.

Cocculus 6 or 30 Made worse by loss of sleep. May want to drink beer.

Nux Vomica 6 or 30 Dizzy and faint in a crowd or in a room with glaring lights. Worse having an empty stomach, or from lack of sleep.

Pulsatilla 6 or 30 Comes on in a warm room and while walking in the open air. Worse while sitting and with menstrual disturbances.

Sulphur 6 or 30 From stooping, being up high, or outdoors.

Voice Loss

See *Hoarseness.*

Vomiting

See *Nausea.*

Whooping Cough (Pertussis)

An infectious disorder occurring mostly in children. It affects the mucous membrane lining of the air passages, and causes frequent attacks of paroxysmal coughing, often ending in vomiting. The incubation period is 7–10 days. It begins with catarrhal symptoms of a cold followed by a spasmodic cough. Always seek professional help, particularly with young babies.

Remedies

Arnica 6 or 30 Child cries before the violent spasmodic cough which causes bloodshot eyes. Worse from exertion of any kind. Chest pain takes the breath away.

Belladonna 6 or 30 Before coughing the child cries and goes red in the face. There is a short, tickling, dry, barking cough which may end in sneezing.

Bryonia 6 or 30 A dry, painful cough which is worse from drinking and eating, taking a deep breath, and coming into a warm room. Patients must sit up and hold or press the chest for relief.

Carbo Veg 6 or 30 Choking cough with vomiting and burning in the chest, worse for cold drinks. Goes blue in the face. Profuse mucus with retching. Craves air, likes to be fanned.

Coccus Cacti 6 or 30 Violent tickling cough ending in vomiting of stringy mucus which hangs from mouth. Face goes purple-red. Cold drinks and cold air bring relief.

Drosera 6 or 30 Feels like a feather tickling the throat. Fits of rapid, deep, barking, incessant cough during which they hold their sides. Begins as soon as head touches the pillow at night.

Ipecac 6 or 30 Child stiffens out and becomes red or blue. Gasps for breath. Incessant, suffocative cough, with nausea. There may be an accompanying nosebleed. Loose rattly cough, but nothing is brought up; or there are copious amounts of foamy mucus.

Pertussin 30 Can be used as a prophylactic. Give 3 doses in 1 week if your child is in contact with whooping cough.

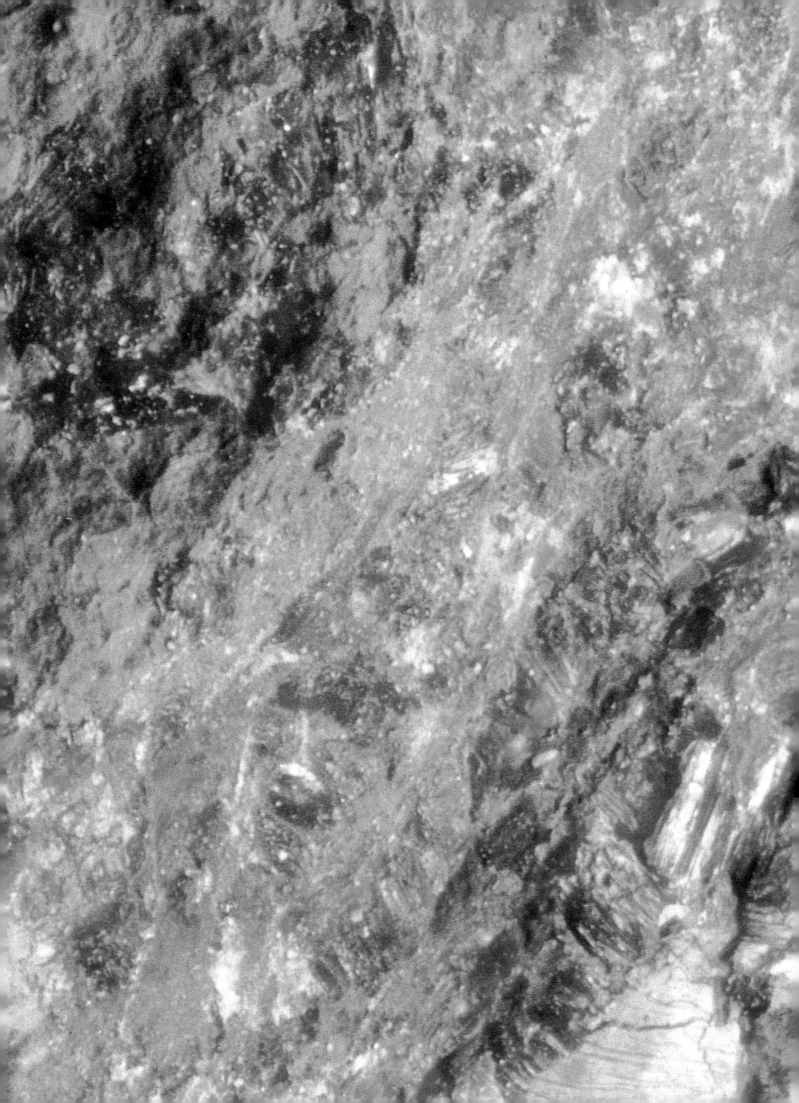

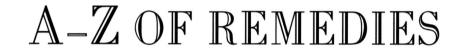

A–Z OF REMEDIES

This selection of the most useful homeopathic medicines for accidents and illness contains details of more than 80 remedies. The name given first is the popular name used by homeopaths, then follows its Latin name, and its common name. The information is set out with a description of the remedy's origins in the mineral world or plant or animal kingdoms, together with a brief history of past usage. Other sub-headings, included where applicable, are as follows:

Characteristic symptoms: *These are like a personal trademark. Even though these symptoms appear in many other remedies, this combination is peculiar to this remedy.*

Areas of application: *Remedies have a vast range of application. The areas given here include a few serious acute illnesses which may require several different remedies to restore the person to health. If improvement is not obtained in a reasonable amount of time, seek the help of a professional homeopath or doctor.*

Pain: *These are the types of pain this remedy covers.*

Worse/better: *The person or their physical body will feel worse or better in the circumstances described.*

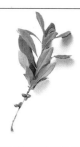
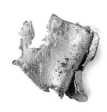
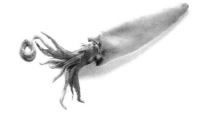

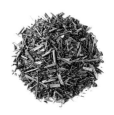

Aconite

Aconitum napellus
Monkshood, Wolfsbane

This perennial plant, with blue helmet-shaped flowers, flourishes in windy mountainous regions and moist pastures in central and southern Europe. It is found in south-west England and South Wales in damp woodland and along the shaded banks of streams. It is thought that Samuel Hahnemann's proving of Aconite (published in 1805) did more to spread the knowledge of homeopathy than any other remedy. In fevers and inflammation, Aconite led the way for a reduction in bloodletting which was popular in medical circles at that time. In its natural state, the plant is deadly poisonous, but it becomes innocuous once it has been diluted and made into a homeopathic remedy. The whole plant is used, gathered when it first flowers.

Characteristic symptoms
Fear, fever and restlessness accompany many symptoms, which are sudden, acute, intense and painful, and have been likened to a storm which disappears as suddenly as it comes. There may be tremendous fear, even with minor ailments. Patients fear they will die, may even predict the time of their death. Afraid to go out of the house. Very high fevers with dry burning heat or drenching sweats with thirst. Chills alternate with heat. Hot red cheeks, or one red, the other pale. Become deathly pale on sitting up in bed. Everything tastes bitter except water. Tingling and numbness which remains after pain has gone. Causes are exposure to cold dry winds – even a draught; heat of the sun; surgical operations and injury; sudden shocks and fright.

Areas of application Use at the beginning of colds, coughs, earache – especially if fever is present. In any situation where fear is predominant, or if it remains a long time after a shock. If menses are delayed after a shock. Retention of urine in a newborn baby after a traumatic birth. Anxiety with palpitations. Asthma, bronchitis, chickenpox, colds, croupy barking cough, cystitis, earache, fainting, hoarseness, measles, mumps, neuralgia, pleurisy, pneumonia, sun headaches, swollen glands, teething, whooping cough.

Pain Unbearable sharp, shooting, burning pains. Tingling and numbness.

Worse At night around midnight; being touched. Cold winds or draughts.

Better Open air.

Aesculus

Aesculus hippocastanum
Horse chestnut tree

This tree was first brought to England from the Balkans in 1616. It is also found in the Himalayas and North America. It was common for people to carry a chestnut in their pocket in the hope that it would prevent or cure piles. And it has been used in Greece and Turkey for the chest complaints of horses, hence its common name – horse chest-nut!

Characteristic symptoms Congestion, engorgement, soreness and throbbing of piles, liver, abdomen. Rectum feels full of small sticks. Piles (purple or blue) which rarely bleed; sharp, shooting pain which goes up the back. Small of the back gives out, especially in pregnancy. Backache after a difficult, large stool, which makes walking almost impossible; agony stooping or rising from sitting.

Areas of application Anal prolapse after stool, lameness during pregnancy, phlebitis, piles.

Pain Sore, burning, shooting, throbbing. Sensation of fullness, little sticks, or a knife.

Worse Rising from sitting, stooping, walking. Pregnancy, menopause.

Better Kneeling, bleeding (piles).

Aethusa

Aethusa cynapium
Fool's parsley

This poisonous plant is a common annual weed in fields, gardens and waste ground and can be mistaken for parsley. The remedy is made from the whole flowering plant.

Characteristic symptoms Teething complaints of babies, especially where they are unable to tolerate milk.

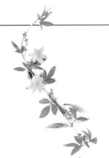
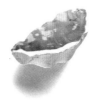
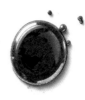
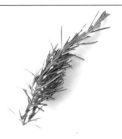

Violent, sudden vomiting of curdled milk immediately after swallowing. Goes limp and falls asleep after vomiting. Wakes hungry and vomits again after feeding. Babies can't hold their head up. Mentally exhausted, unable to concentrate or think – caused by overstudying.

Areas of application Projectile vomiting in teething babies. Violent vomiting in pregnancy. Inability to focus mind, e.g. in studying.

Pain Violent, lancinating pains.

Worse Milk. Warmth. Hot weather. Teething. Over-exertion.

Better Walking in open air.

Agaricus
Agaricus muscarius
Fly agaric, Toadstool

This well-known poisonous mushroom is found under birch trees in the autumn and in pine woods. In the past it was used as a fly poison. It can cause delirium and intoxication, and sometimes death.

Characteristic symptoms
Sensation as if pierced by cold needles. Painful twitchings, then the part becomes stiff and cold, as if frozen. Burning, itching, redness and swelling. Itching moves around on scratching. Clumsy, drops things.

Areas of application Bunions, chilblains, frostbite.

Pain Like ice-cold needles, stitching pains.

Worse Cold air, playing in the snow, mountain climbing, skiing. Sunlight.

Better Warmth and sitting by a fire.

Allium Cepa
Common red onion

Onions have been used in the past to absorb the poisons of contagious diseases such as the plague and give protection from evil spirits. The juice is said to increase sperm, kill worms and soothe scalds and burns. A raw onion eaten just before bedtime can help sleeplessness. The effects of cutting an onion are well known – streaming nose and eyes with burning and smarting pains.

Characteristic symptoms Increased secretions from the eyes and nose, like those of the common cold. Frequent sneezing, with watery discharge which burns the nose and upper lip, but the eye discharge is bland and doesn't burn (see Euphrasia, which has the opposite effect). Tickling in the throat with incessant cough – as if larynx is split. Holds throat.

Areas of application
Catarrhal headache, common cold, hayfever, tickly cough.

Common red onion

Worse On entering a warm room (nasal symptoms). Getting feet wet. May be one-sided, e.g. one nostril runs more.

Better In cool open air, except cough.

Anacardium
Anacardium orientale
Malacca nut, Marking nut

This tree was known in Arabia over a thousand years ago. The remedy is made from a black juice which is found between the outer, black, heart-shaped shell and the sweet kernel inside. In India the juice has been used to mark linen, hence the name marking nut.

Characteristic symptoms Eating relieves many of the complaints – nervous dyspepsia, weak feeling with emptiness in stomach, nausea of pregnancy – but they return once the food has been digested (contrast Nux Vomica, which feels worse for two or three hours after eating and better once the food has been digested). Sensation of a plug in various parts or a band around the body. Loss of memory and confidence. May swear a lot.

Areas of application Morning sickness of pregnancy. Weak digestion.

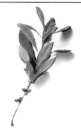
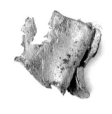
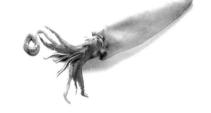

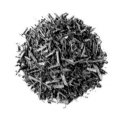

Nervous exhaustion from overstudy. Poor memory. Lack of self-confidence. Useful in examinations.

Pain Penetrating like a plug. Constricting like a band.

Worse Mental strain, anger, in the morning, strong smells.

Better Eating.

Ant Crud
Antimonium crudum
Sulphide of antimony

A grey-black powder found in nature. Much information was acquired from the slow poisoning experienced by those mining it. Pigs used to be fed on it to fatten them up, and a powdered form was used to make kohl. In its crystalline form it is known as stibnite and can be useful with disorders of the stomach and oesophagus, and can relieve stiffness and rigidity.

Characteristic symptoms An angry child – children cannot bear to be touched or looked at and tell you to go away (Chamomilla children call you back). There may be a ravenous appetite which easily leads to digestive problems from overloading the stomach. Sudden vomiting in babies after taking milk (breast or bottle), who may want to feed again immediately. Desire for acids and pickles which aggravate the digestion. Appetite does not return after illness. Thickly coated white tongue as if whitewashed. A strange absence of pain where normally expected. Scabby crusts and cracks in nostrils and corners of the mouth; injured nails remain split and skin thickens around them; corns and veruccas on soles of feet.

Areas of application Disturbed digestion. Sudden vomiting after eating. Vomiting during measles and pregnancy, and from getting overheated. Callosities on hands and feet. Cracks in skin.

Sulphide of antimony

Pain An absence of pain where it would normally be expected.

Worse Overeating. Acids, vinegar, sour wine and pork. Swimming or washing in cold water. Heat and hot sunny weather.

Better In the open air. Moist warmth.

Ant Tart
Antimonium tartaricum
Tartar emetic

This poison was popularly used to purge the contents of stomach and bowel, but often led to death when it was absorbed into the body.

Characteristic symptoms Drowsiness, or yawning, and a cold clammy sweat with many complaints. Waves of nausea and weakness, with thick white coating on tongue. In respiratory complaints, the chest sounds full up with phlegm which can be heard rattling from a distance, but because of weakness there is great difficulty in bringing it up. Children want to be carried upright. Their anger brings on suffocative coughing fits. A dry, teasing cough may come on before a rash develops (e.g. in measles). Skin eruptions of bluish pustules. Crave apples, sharp-tasting things; dislike milk.

Areas of application Chickenpox, measles, whooping cough. Coughs which come on during teething. Bronchitis, pneumonia. Loose, rattling cough which may end in vomiting, as if drowning in own secretions. Can be used in cases of near drowning. Nausea and vomiting of pregnancy.

Worse Sour things; lying down; being touched or looked at; overheated.

Better Sitting up; vomiting; coughing up phlegm.

Apis
Apis mellifica
Honey bee

The remedy is made either from the whole bee, or from its venom. In folk medicine, bees have been used to cure dropsy and to help newborn babies pass urine. It is therefore a remedy which could be considered for water retention.

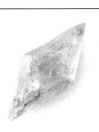
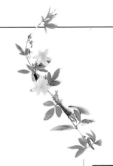
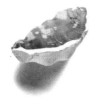

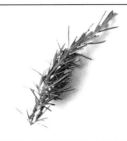

Characteristic symptoms Fidgety, fussy and hard to please. Jealous nature. Awkward, drops things. Debility as if worked too hard. Dreams of being busy. Longs to sleep but too restless. Rapid development of symptoms. Pain comes suddenly. Screams in sleep or cries out in pain. Puffy swellings anywhere, particularly eyelids and under eyes. Shiny, rosy red skin. Drowsy and thirstless with fever. Air hunger; panting with each breath as if the last. Worse for heat in any form.

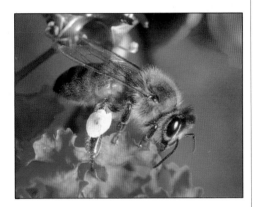

Honey bee

Areas of application Abscess, asthma, boils, carbuncles, conjunctivitis, cystitis, earache, insect bites, nettlerash, scarlet fever, shingles, stings, styes. Severe allergic reactions to stings, certain foods or medicines (*see* Shock and Collapse, page 43). Tonsillitis, water retention.

Pain Burning like hot needles, stinging, smarting. Bruised soreness.

Worse Hot room, hot weather. Hot drinks. Touch, even of hair.

Better Cool air. Cool bathing. Cold drinks. Movement.

Arg Nit
Argenticum nitricum
Nitrate of silver

Until relatively recently, diluted silver nitrate was routinely dropped into the eyes of newborn babies with the intention of preventing the spread of gonorrhoea, which is known to cause blindness. It was also used to cauterize wounds and has been known to turn skin permanently blue if accidentally swallowed.

Characteristic symptoms Always in a hurry, impulsive, acts before thinking. Impatient. Anticipates things will not go well. Extreme anxiety with trembling, flatulence and diarrhoea, which is noisy and explosive and comes on immediately after eating or drinking. There is a fondness for sweet food, which causes diarrhoea.

Areas of application Conjunctivitis. Sticky discharge from eyes, especially in newborn babies. Fear, anxiety, anticipation. Diarrhoea before an important event such as driving test, interview, examinations, public speaking, flying.

Pain Splinter-like, sharp, shoots like lightning.

Worse In a warm room or enclosed space such as an aircraft. Looking down. Crowds. Warmth or stuffiness. Mental strain. Sugar.

Better Cool open air. The company of people.

Arnica
Arnica montana
Leopard's bane, Mountain tobacco

Another name for this plant is 'fallkraut' (fall-herb) which gives a clue to its use – it is the main accident remedy. It grows in mountainous regions all over the world and has an ancient reputation for healing injuries.

Characteristic symptoms When someone has been injured and obviously needs help, Arnica is always the first remedy to give to reduce the impact of shock, haemorrhage and bruising. The shock of an accident can cut a person off from what's going on in the physical body; in Arnica this may be shown as a denial that anything is wrong. There is fear of being touched, because of the pain. In acute illness they grumble that the bed feels too hard (even if it is soft) and this causes restlessness because they cannot get comfortable. Taste of bad eggs in mouth. Head feels hot, body cold. Swellings with discoloration (compare Symphytum). Arnica helps blood clots to be absorbed.

Areas of application Shock, trauma, bruising, violence to mind or body. Any accident or operation, minor and major. Bleeding of small wounds such as a cut from shaving. Nosebleed from blowing the nose, coughing, or during fever. Over-exertion. Sprains and strains. Hoarse voice from overstraining. In pregnancy when the baby's movements are unbearably

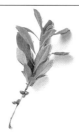
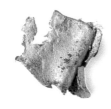
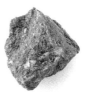
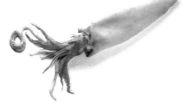
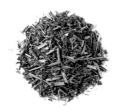

painful. Unable to pass urine after giving birth because of bruising. Threatened miscarriage after a fall. Palpitations after exertion. Crops of small boils. Phlebitis. Septic conditions. Violent coughs, whooping cough. Children cry before cough comes on. Influenza. Typhoid fever. Insect stings, splinters.

CAUTION: Arnica ointment should never be applied to broken skin as it may cause a rash.

Pain Sore, aching and bruised. Stitching chest pains take the breath away.

Worse Slightest touch.

Better Lying down and with head low.

Arsenicum
Arsenicum album
White oxide of metallic arsenic

Arsenic is a metallic element found in many minerals and needs no introduction as a poison. It has been used for criminal purposes for hundreds of years. It has also been widely used in the dyeing, wallpaper, paint and food industries. People living and working in mountainous areas have taken it to 'strengthen' their muscles, which enabled them to climb more easily with heavy loads. It is still used in tonic drinks in some parts of the world. Taken in small doses regularly, it will accumulate in the body and may cause thickening and darkening of the skin.

Characteristic symptoms Weakness out of all proportion to symptoms. Extremely anxious, nervous and restless. Sudden great weakness and collapse from very slight causes. Fears being alone. Feels the cold but also wants fresh air. Anxiety over health is a big preoccupation. Fussy people who are quick to criticize. One unusual symptom is that burning pains are relieved by heat. Very thirsty for frequent sips of cold water, which may then be vomited immediately. Colds, which descend to the chest, have a watery discharge which burns the skin under the nose. In asthma the face may be covered with cold sweat. Throat is extremely dry, swollen, ulcerated and burning, all relieved by hot drinks. Children may restlessly change beds several times in the night.

Areas of application
Abscess, boils. Asthma. Burns. Cold sores. Colds. Dandruff. Fever. Food poisoning. Gangrene. Headaches. Mouth ulcers. Shingles. Sinuses. Sleeplessness. Swollen throat. Vomiting and diarrhoea.

Pain Burning like fire or hot needles.

Worse Just after midnight to 2 a.m. Periodically, e.g. yearly. At weekends when relaxing from work. Vegetables and watery fruits. Cold food and drink.

Better Heat, hot drinks and food. Milk.

Moving about. Company. Sitting upright. Cold flannel or walking in open air (headache).

Baptisia
Baptisia tinctoria
Wild indigo

This plant grows wild in North America and until a synthetic version

Wild indigo *was introduced it was used to dye fabric a blue-violet colour. It has been used as an antiseptic for dressing wounds, especially those accompanied by fever. The remedy is made from the root and bark.*

Characteristic symptoms There is a drowsy, almost drunken look with a dusky red complexion. Symptoms closely resemble typhoid fever. Septic state of the body. Weakness comes on rapidly. Soreness, aching and heaviness in muscles all over body. Sense of duality in delirium; parts of the body feel separated or scattered. Confused. Falls asleep while speaking. Offensive discharges and odour of the body. Complains that the bed feels too hard (like Arnica). Tongue feels burnt. Dark red mouth, swollen throat, which may be ulcerated.

Areas of application Appendicitis. Dysentery. Gastric flu. Influenza. Low fever. Mumps. Relatively pain-free sore

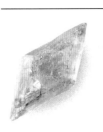 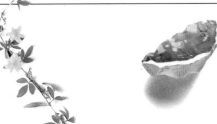 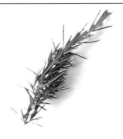

throat. Tonsillitis. Typhoid fever. Antidotes bad effects of anti-typhoid serum.

Pain Sore, aching with heaviness, numbness.

Worse Humid heat.

Better Sweating.

Belladonna
Atropa belladonna
Deadly nightshade

Poisoning causes congestion of blood to the head and face, with throbbing or bursting pains. This in turn leads to excitement and restlessness. Eyes dilate and stare, and become extremely sensitive to light. Death occurs in severe cases. The remedy is made from the whole plant as it begins to flower.

Characteristic symptoms Symptoms come and go suddenly. Congestion, especially of the blood vessels in the head, causing throbbing headaches. Wild or excited condition. Burning heat, bright redness, throbbing and dryness, with restlessness. Hot head with cold arms and legs. Thirstless with fever. Eyes very sensitive to light. Delerious – sees monsters and doesn't recognize familiar people. A barking cough. Desires lemonade. Discharges (e.g. blood during menstruation) feel hot. Strawberry tongue.

Areas of application Childbirth. Children's fevers. Croup. Earache.

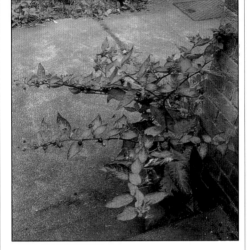
Deadly nightshade

Glandular swellings. Headache. Influenza. Measles. Menstruation. Mumps. Pleurisy. Pneumonia. Scarlet Fever. Sore throat. Sunstroke. Tonsillitis. Toothache.

Pain Throbbing, burning, shooting, stabbing. Cramp. Violent dragging-down feeling. Severe neuralgic pain.

Worse Touch. Light. Noise. Being jarred (having the bed knocked). Sun. Draughts to the head. Haircut. Washing the hair. During the night.

Better Bending backwards. Warmth.

Common daisy

Bellis Perennis
Common daisy

One of the most popular habitats of this wild flower is the garden lawn, where it will survive being cut regularly by a lawn-mower. It is

also known as wound-wort or bruise-wort and has the ability to bounce back after being trodden on. It is similar to Arnica in its sphere of action but works on a deeper level. The remedy is made from the whole fresh plant.

Characteristic symptoms Trauma to abdomen and pelvic organs, especially after surgery and childbirth if Arnica does not give relief. Septic wounds. Stagnation in veins. Injuries to nerves with intense soreness. Fullness in the breasts and uterus. Difficulty walking in pregnancy. Wakes up too early and can't get back to sleep. Backache from hard physical work, such as gardening.

Areas of application Abdominal surgery. After forceps delivery. Arthritis. Boils. Caesarean. Catarrh. Coughs. D & C (womb scrape). Diarrhoea. Falls on to the coccyx (tail bone). Fatigue and overwork. Pregnancy. Rheumatism. Symptoms that develop after suddenly getting chilled on a hot day. Varicose veins.

Pain Bruised. Sore. Aching.

Worse Touch. After getting wet or taking cold drinks or ices when overheated.

Better Cold compresses applied to painful part.

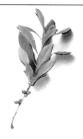
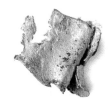
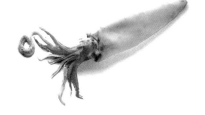

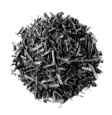

Bryonia

Bryonia alba

Wild hops

The plant is extremely poisonous and children have died within a few hours of eating the berries. The remedy is made from a tincture of the root, gathered before the plant flowers.

Characteristic symptoms An irritable person who wants to be left alone. Prefers damp weather. Dryness of the mucous membranes. Movement of any kind aggravates, even talking. Holds the part that hurts: holds the sides or head during cough, or prefers to lie on the painful breast in mastitis to keep it still. Sitting up in bed can bring on vomiting. Children don't want to be carried. Symptoms develop slowly. Sharp stitching pain in chest or at the lower angle of the right shoulder blade. Lips feel burnt.

Areas of application Asthma. Bronchitis. Constipation. Dry cough. Feverish colds which may descend to the chest. Gastro-enteritis. Influenza. Joint injuries when Arnica hasn't brought relief. Joint pain. Mastitis. Measles. Pneumonia. Pleurisy. Rheumatism. Stiff neck. Teething. Whooping cough.

Pain Stitching, bursting. Heaviness.

Worse Deep breathing. In a hot room. Dry weather. Hot weather. Slightest movement. Sitting up. Touch.

Better Pressure and lying on the painful part to keep it still. Cool, open air. Being quiet or alone. Cloudy, damp days.

Calc Carb

Calcarea carbonica

Calcium carbonate, Carbonate of lime

Oyster shell

The metallic element calcium is widely found in various compounds in minerals (chalk), animals and plants. Calcium salts give us our skeletal framework. The remedy is made from the inner layer of the oyster shell. A person who needs this in homeopathic potency is described as an oyster without a shell – flabby, plump and pale.

Characteristic symptoms Sour-smelling, cold sweat during sleep, on the head, neck and chest, or from slightest effort. Cold, clammy feet. Lethargic babies who are late walking and teething, happy just to sit; their pillow is soaked with sweat after sleep. Chilly, inactive people. Shortness of breath on climbing stairs. Colds go to the chest. Cramps in calf muscles when stretching legs in bed. In breastfeeding there is too much milk, which constantly leaks out. Constipated but this doesn't seem to bother them. Crave eggs.

Areas of application Breastfeeding. Bronchial catarrh in teething children. Chilblains. Croup. Earache. Glandular swellings. Lingering thick, yellow catarrh with loss of smell. Painful, swollen breasts before menses. Strains; mental strain.

Pain Cramp. Throbbing.

Worse Cold weather. Damp air. Washing or swimming in cold water. Going up stairs. Milk. Exerting themselves mentally or physically.

Better Dry weather. Warmth.

Calc Fluor

Calcarea fluorica

Fluoride of lime, Fluorspar

This mineral is found as a crystal throughout the world. Its qualities as a remedy are of great use throughout pregnancy.

Characteristic symptoms It helps muscles and connective tissue to stretch and is needed in the surface of bones and tooth enamel. Without it a sluggish condition develops, leading to things such as piles and varicose veins. Helps remove scar tissue after operations.

Areas of application Bearing-down pains in the lower back, with a tired

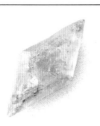
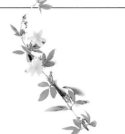
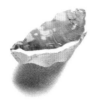
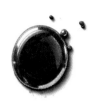
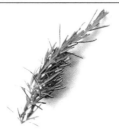

feeling. Piles. Pregnancy. Stony-hard glands and tonsils. Varicose veins. X-ray burns. Use if Rhus Tox doesn't work for symptoms which feel better once the initial painful movement has been made (e.g. in backache).

Worse Humid conditions, and cold, damp weather. On beginning to move.

Better Massage and warmth. Continued movement.

Calc Phos
Calcarea phosphorica
Phosphate of lime

Calcium phosphate is a mineral salt which is needed in the body for the nutrition of blood cells and the formation of bones and teeth. It is therefore very important for children and in pregnancy.

Characteristic symptoms Children who grow fast and always seem tired. They are restless, discontented and always want to be somewhere else. Headaches from overstudying – pain near the sutures of the skull. Useful when taken during convalescence after an acute illness. Child loses breath on being lifted up.

Areas of application Anaemia after acute illness. Broken bones. Pregnancy. At puberty when menstruation starts and the flow is

heavy. Recurring teeth problems, teething babies. Swollen glands.

Pain Burning.

Worse Changes in the weather. Wet weather. Being lifted up.

Better Lying down. Warm, dry days.

Calc Sulph
Calcarea sulphurica
Gypsum, Plaster of Paris

Gypsum

Gypsum is found in a crystallized state – alabaster – or in the form of a soft chalky stone which when heated becomes the fine white powder known as plaster of Paris.

Characteristic symptoms
Unhealthy skin that will not heal. Wounds and spots which have begun to discharge pus, with no end in sight. Discharges are yellow, thick and lumpy, possibly blood-streaked. (Compare Hepar Sulph, which is worse from any exposure to cold air.)

Areas of application
Abscesses. Acne. Blood purifier. Boils. Burns and scalds. Carbuncles. Chilblains. Colds. Earache. Tonsillitis. Calc Sulph will help in these situations when there is a catarrhal or

pus-filled discharge, which may be blood-streaked.

Worse Draughts. Getting wet. Change of weather.

Better Open air.

Calendula
Calendula officinalis
Marigold

This is a hardy annual plant with flowers of different shades of yellow and orange. At dawn the flower opens with the rising sun and closes at sunset. Its response to clouds is also to close. The Latin name Calendula was given to it after the Romans noticed that the Marigold was usually in bloom on the first day, or calends, of every month. It was used by surgeons to prevent the spread of septic conditions in war wounds in the 1800s, and as a hot fomentation in pneumonia and to strengthen the heart. The remedy is made from a tincture of the leaves and flowers. It is mostly used externally, but may also be taken in pill form. Information given in this book applies to the external use of Calendula, either as an ointment or a diluted tincture unless otherwise mentioned.

Marigold

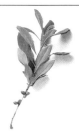
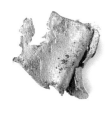
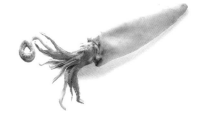

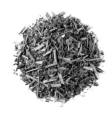

Characteristic symptoms Lacerated and suppurating wounds which may be slow to heal. It revitalizes injured parts, preventing the formation of pus, creating a new covering over a wound. Pain is out of proportion to the injury.

CAUTION: Clean wounds very thoroughly, because Calendula helps close the skin extremely fast, and grit, etc, could be sealed inside.

Areas of application Any open wound. Abscess. Burns. Carbuncle. During labour and birth to soothe perineum. Gangrene. Haemorrhages – after tooth extraction, torn perineum or episiotomy during birth. Jaundice (internally). Offensive discharge after forceps delivery (take Calendula 6 or 30 internally, as well as gently sponging the perineum – *see* Labour, page 36, and Surgery, page 45). Tetanus (internally).

Pain Excessive, out of all proportion to the injury.

Worse Damp, cloudy days.

Cantharis
Cantharis vesicatoria
Spanish fly

The remedy is made from a beetle which inhabits Spain, Italy, Sicily and southern Russia. It was once in widespread use as an agent to cause blisters on the skin as a means of relieving congestion in organs of the body.

Spanish fly

Characteristic symptoms Irritation and violent inflammation, particularly of urinary and sexual organs. Rapid onset. Urine burns and scalds, bloody. Unbearable urge to urinate but only a few drops are passed. Burning thirst, but drinking aggravates.

Areas of application After episiotomy. Blisters from sunburn. Burns and scalds. Cystitis. Yellow fever.

Pain Violent burning, cutting, stabbing or smarting. Rawness.

Worse During and after urinating. Cold drinks, coffee.

Better Warmth, rest and rubbing.

Carbo Veg
Carbo vegetabilis
Wood charcoal

Charcoal has deodorant and disinfectant properties and contains oxygen which is released when it comes into contact with decomposing matter. This remedy is usually made from charcoal obtained from poplar, beech or birch wood.

Characteristic symptoms Flatulence, weakness and craving for air are the leading symptoms, accompanied by a sluggish mental and physical condition, and burning pains. The processes of decay and putrefaction run throughout this remedy. Slow digestion with excessive accumulation of gas; feel better once gas is passed up or down. Weakness shows in their lack of reaction after a shock or attack. They want moving air around them, so may ask to be fanned, but with this they are often icy cold, with a hot head. Very slow recovery from illness.

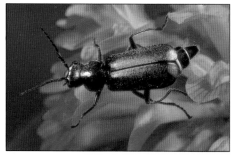

Wood charcoal

Areas of application Acidity. Acne. Asthma. Bed sores. Burns. Carbuncles. Chilblains. Colic. Collapse. Food poisoning. Gangrene. Haemorrhage (after the shock of surgery). Haemorrhoids. Indigestion. Labour and pregnancy. Nosebleed on straining at stool. Septic states. Varicose veins. Whooping cough. Yellow fever.

Pain Burning.

Worse Tight clothing. Lying down (flatulence). Decaying meat and fish. Rich, fatty food. Butter. Milk. Ice water. Warmth. Going from a warm room to cold air (cough). Evening.

Better Belching. Cool moving air.

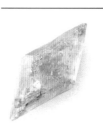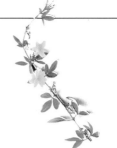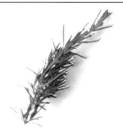

Carbolic Acid

Carbolicum acidum

This is a powerful antiseptic. During its use in surgery in the past, it has poisoned patients and surgeons and has thereby given valuable information for its homeopathic uses.

Characteristic symptoms Collapse, sometimes coming on after a severe allergic reaction to the stings of poisonous spiders, scorpions or snakes. Intense pains which come and go suddenly. The sense of smell becomes very acute, which is a leading symptom of this remedy. There is paleness around the nose and mouth. Gasps for breath. Numbness and twitching. Urine turns dark green. Discharges smell rotten.

Areas of application Bites and stings from poisonous insects or snakes leading to collapse. Old or ulcerated burns with an offensive discharge.

Pain Burning, pricking like needles.

Worse Warm room and cold air.

Castor Equi

Horse's thumbnail

The rudimentary thumbnail of the horse is a small, flat, oval horn, wrinkled on its surface, breaking off in scales, which grows on the inner side of the leg above the fetlock. The scales are used for homeopathic purposes. It is a very ancient remedy.

Characteristic symptoms Excessively tender, sore, cracked nipples. There may be ulceration.

Areas of application Cracked, sore nipples. Ulcerated nipples.

Pain Sore. Tender.

Worse During breastfeeding. Touch of clothes.

Blue cohosh

Caulophyllum

Caulophyllum thalictroides

Blue cohosh, Squaw root

Squaw root was widely used by Native Americans to ease the pains of childbirth. Homeopaths also use Caulophyllum frequently in situations described below, and may give it towards the end of pregnancy, if indicated.

Characteristic symptoms Gynaecological and rheumatic symptoms. Rheumatism, particularly of the small joints. Vaginal discharge (leucorrhoea) in young girls. Repeated miscarriages from weakness of womb. False labour pains. Can be used to prevent a long, painful labour. Contractions are too painful, irregular, ineffectual, go to the groin, or disappear because of the exhaustion of a long labour. Prolonged vaginal discharge after birth. Nervous excitement – sleepless and restless, with internal trembling. After birth uterine muscles do not contract properly through lack of tone. This is a potentially dangerous situation as it may lead to haemorrhage.

Areas of application Exhaustion in a long, painful labour: 'No progress'. False labour pains. Rigid cervix. Rheumatism of small joints. Atony of womb after labour.

Pain Erratic – flies about. Bearing down. Pricking like needles (cervix). Cramp.

Worse Labour. Pregnancy. Open air.

Causticum

Potassium hydrate

This substance was created by Hahnemann from burnt lime (marble) and bisulphate of potash.

Characteristic symptoms People are oversympathetic and suffer long after someone they were fond of moves away or dies. They may spend many hours looking after a sick relative, with consequent loss of sleep which weakens them. Children are frightened to go to bed alone. Paralysis and weakness in the throat and chest muscles which prevents coughing deeply enough to bring up phlegm, or they can't spit it out. Incessant cough from a tickle in the throat which is

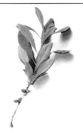
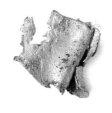
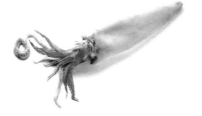

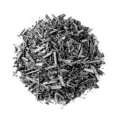

better from sipping cold water. Children wet the bed in the first few hours of sleep. Stress incontinence – leaky bladder on coughing, sneezing or blowing nose. Unable to pass urine after childbirth or surgery. Restless legs in bed. Rheumaticky pains which are better in damp weather (unusual). A remedy for deep burns and their long-term effects.

Areas of application After episiotomy. Bedwetting. Bronchitis. Coughs. Cystitis. Deep burns. Facial neuralgia (if Aconite doesn't relieve). Hoarseness (of singers). Joints. Lead poisoning. Pregnancy and labour. Rheumatism. Weak bladder.

Pain Scraping rawness. Sore. Burning. Cramps. Electric shocks (legs).

German chamomile

Worse Dry, cold wind. Evening at twilight. Speaking (cough). Coughing, sneezing, blowing nose (bladder).

Better Damp, rainy weather. Warmth of bed. Cold drinks (cough).

Chamomilla

Matricaria chamomilla
German chamomile

The remedy is made from German chamomile, as distinct from Roman chamomile. There is conflicting information in herbal books about these plants, which says something about one of its chief symptoms – that of contrariness! Its ability to be 'abusive' is also illustrated by a quote from the English herbalist Culpeper, who did not think too highly of German chamomile – he called it a 'hateful weed'. There was much discussion over the merits of the different plants. In Hahnemann's day physicians referred to it as a 'vulgar domestic remedy' – they were unfamiliar with the latent power waiting to be released with homeopathic potentization. Instances of mild poisoning occurred from its over-use, which carries on today with the regular drinking of chamomile tea: unusual irritability and sleeplessness may be pointers to this. On compost heaps it assists calcium in the decomposing process.

Characteristic symptoms Can't bear anything, or anyone. Pain is unbearable and drives them mad; they demand that you immediately do something about it. Extremely angry and abusive, or spiteful, which causes many symptoms. Impossible to please. Contrariness. Children demand things and immediately throw them down and want something else. They insist on being carried. In fever, one cheek red and hot, the other pale and cold. Breastfed babies may develop colic after mother's anger. Teething babies have diarrhoea looking like chopped egg and spinach, smelling of rotten eggs.

Areas of application Asthma. Colic. Convulsions in teething babies from anger. Cough. Cramp. Croup. Diarrhoea. Earache. Excitement. Fainting. Fevers. Labour. Mastitis. Menstrual pain. Miscarriage (from anger). Pain. Tearfulness. Teething. Toothache. Whooping cough.

Pain Burning. Smarting. Cutting. Throbbing. Bursting. Neuralgic and rheumatic. Cramp. Pains with numbness. Hot sweat with pain.

Worse Pain. Touch. Being looked at. Lying in bed. Night. Around 9 p.m. Teething. Coffee.

Better Being carried. Warmth (the person). Cold (local parts). Ice-cold water (toothache).

China

China officinalis
Cinchona bark, Peruvian bark

In 1638 the Countess of Chinchon (in Spain), wife of the Viceroy of Peru, was cured of fever from the bark of this tree, which contains quinine. The local Peruvians felt the tree to be guarded by special gods and would not let it be touched. In spite of this, a huge industry eventually grew in the export of the bark to Europe – up to

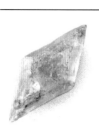 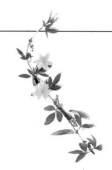 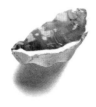 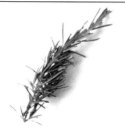

500,000 pounds annually – where it was used to treat malaria and other fevers. Poisoning from its over-use, which became widespread, was known as cinchonism. In 1790 Samuel Hahnemann took the bark himself as an experiment. The results he obtained led him to the discovery of the Law of Cure (see pages 8–9, Principles of Homeopathy), and this experience formed the foundation on which he was to build the reputation of homeopathy.

Characteristic symptoms Thin anaemic blood. Weakness and exhaustion from heavy losses of body fluids via breast milk, sweating, vomiting, diarrhoea, or from emotional worries. Loss of appetite which returns on beginning to eat. Full up very quickly while eating. Slow digestion (compare Carbo Veg) especially after a late supper. Bitter taste in mouth. Post-operative gas pains – no relief from passing (opposite of Carbo Veg), or it remains stuck. Pale face with blue rings round eyes. In labour where there is heavy blood loss in the mother, and the baby's life is subsequently threatened. Wounds become black and gangrenous. Add a few drops to drinking water when travelling (see below).

Areas of application Anaemia. Breastfeeding. Childbirth. Colic. Exhaustion. Fainting. Flatulent bloating. Gangrene. Haemorrhage. Indigestion. Stimulates appetite. Surgery. Weakness.

Pain Bursting. Throbbing. Neuralgic. Sore. Knife-like.

Worse Loss of body fluids. On alternate days; periodically. Touch. Milk, tea, fruit, contaminated water, meat, fish. Cold. Draughts.

Better Loose clothes. Bending double. Hard pressure. Warmth.

Cimicifuga
Actea racemosa
Black cohosh

A perennial plant which grows in Canada and the USA and is well known among Native American tribes. The remedy is made from the roots and is particularly useful in labour.

Characteristic symptoms Over-sensitive to pain and noise. In labour, talks through contractions, fidgety and excitable. Gloomy, pessimistic, 'I can't do it', as if she'll go mad. Pains constantly change place or fly from side to side, or shoot up or down the thighs. Slow labour with nervous shivers, trembling legs. Head feels as if the top would fly off or as if hot or cold air were blowing on it.

Areas of application Nausea in pregnancy. Labour. After-pains. Lochia suppressed. Headache. Menses.

Pain Violent pains change place or go from side to side. Shooting. Aching. Sore. Bruised.

Worse Menstruation. During childbirth. Damp, cold air. Sitting.

Better Warmth. Open air. Eating. Continued motion.

Cocculus
Cocculus indicus
Fish berry, India berry

This climbing shrub is found in India and the Far East. Its name means bitter poison and it has been used since ancient times to stupefy fish to make them easier to catch. It was also used in the brewing industry to enhance the intoxifying properties of beer. The remedy is made from the powdered seeds.

Characteristic symptoms Paralysis and weakness. Confusion as if drunk. Travel sickness. Vertigo with nausea and faintness – worse for any movement, even lifting the head. Too weak to hold the head up. Hollow, empty feeling – in head, abdomen, chest. Overstrain from lack of sleep, people who lose sleep while caring for the sick or who work night shifts. Headaches at the start of menses. Abdomen bloated as if full of sharp stones. Drowsiness in labour. Desire for beer.

Areas of application Childbirth. Hangover. Headaches. Overstrain – mental or physical. Painful menstrual colic with weakness. Sleep loss. Travel sickness. Vertigo with fainting and nausea.

Pain Cramps. Spasms like electric shocks.

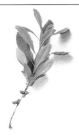
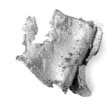

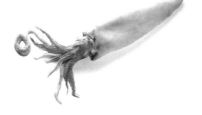
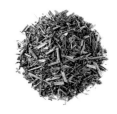

Worse Motion of cars, boats, etc. Loss of sleep. All food and drink. Touch. Cold open air. At menses.

Better Lying on side. In a room.

Coccus Cacti
Cochineal

The natural habitat of the insect Coccus cacti is the prickly pear cactus of Central America. Until recently it was used as a food colouring.

Characteristic symptoms Catarrhal states of the mucous membranes, throat and chest. Irritation of throat causes cough, retching, vomiting. Violent internal itching. Unbearable tickly cough which leads to vomiting of clear ropy mucus, with purple-red face. Constant clearing of throat leads to more coughing and retching. Cough worse brushing teeth. Tongue burns like pepper.

Areas of application Bronchitis. Cough. Whooping cough.

Pain Burning like pepper.

Worse Heat. Lying down. Cold. Brushing teeth.

Better Cold drinks (cough). Washing in cold water.

Coffea
Coffea crudea
Coffee, Mocha bean

Coffee drinking first flourished in Ethiopia many centuries ago. One of its uses was to induce wakefulness during moments of prayer but its reputation changed as its popularity increased and it became linked with dancing and singing. In the seventeenth century, when coffee arrived in Europe, there was a strong reaction from the English clergy, who associated its black colour with the devil. Drinking black coffee can antidote many poisons, especially narcotics. But it has also been known to damage the subtle energy fields around the body and spoil many homeopathic remedies.

Coffee

Characteristic symptoms Over-stimulated mental states. Nerves are over-sensitive. Children become excited at the thought of a forthcoming event and cannot sleep. Restlessness, with laughing and crying, or a pleasant surprise gives them a shock. They wake up at the slightest sound. Pain is unbearable, often with a fear of death. Severe pains in labour, or after-pains. Nervous palpitations after excitement or a surprise. Toothache which is relieved by holding ice-cold water in the mouth. Toothache during menses. Hearing and vision are more acute than usual.

Areas of application Antidotes some drugs. Childbirth. Convulsions in teething children. Excitement. Fainting. Low pain threshold. Neuralgia. Palpitations. Sleeplessness. Toothache.

Pain Unbearable, with fear of death.

Worse Touch. Noise. Smells. Night. Open air. Excitement.

Better Warmth. Lying down. Sleep. Cold drinks (toothache). Pressure.

Colocynth
Colocynthis
Bitter apple, Bitter cucumber

The fruit of a species of cucumber growing in the Mediterranean region and known as far back as 500 BC, it was once used as a powerful purgative. In homeopathic preparation its use is for severe colic.

Characteristic symptoms The main areas affected are the abdominal, facial and sciatic nerves. Many complaints are caused by anger. The person is touchy and easily offended. Abdomen feels as if intestines are squeezed between stones. Screams or faints and vomits with pain. In colic, babies prefer to lie on the stomach. Cramps in hips, better lying on the painful side. Diarrhoea from pain or anger. A useful antidote to lead poisoning.

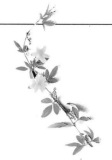

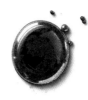
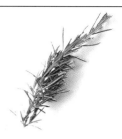

Areas of application After-effects of surgery on orifices, e.g. anus, urethra. Colic. Painful menses. Suppressed menses, or lochia, from indignation. Neuralgia. Sciatica.

Pain Waves of pain – cutting, pinching, tearing, throbbing, cramping, shooting – as if an iron band gripped them.

Worse From emotions, anger. Lying on painless side. Any food or drink, except coffee or tobacco. Night.

Better Hard pressure. Bending double. Heat. Rest. Lying on the painful side.

Crotalus Horridus
Rattlesnake

Venom from the rattlesnake is one of many used in the homeopathic pharmacopoeia, and illustrates again how something poisonous can be transformed, via the dilution process, into an agent for healing. The remedy is made from a solution of the snake venom which has been dried and preserved in glycerine.

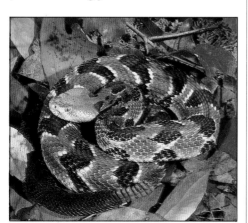

Rattlesnake

Characteristic symptoms It acts on the blood, the heart and the liver. It can be used where there is severe nervous shock. Tissues rapidly decompose and become septic and putrid. The skin can show any colour but a dark bluish colour is common. Breath and secretions from body smell mouldy. Saliva and sweat may be bloody. Haemorrhages ooze dark, thin blood. Dreams of the dead.

Areas of application Haemorrhage. Septic states – abscesses, boils, bites, stings, tonsils, stomach ulcers, gangrene. Yellow fever, blackwater fever.

Pain Burning.

Worse Lying on the right side. Falling asleep (horrible dreams). In the spring. Yearly.

Better Movement.

Cuprum
Cuprum metallicum
Copper

Copper, a red-coloured metal, is mined in many countries of the world. Although it is an essential nutrient and is found in all tissues of the body, it also has the potential to poison those who work closely with it. It has been used medicinally in the past for treating ulcers and in the food industry as a colorant.

Characteristic symptoms Copper is known for its spasmodic effects. It

causes violent cramps and convulsions and is therefore useful for infants with convulsions prompted by teething. Violent cough, loses breath, goes stiff. Convulsions, beginning with jerking in fingers and toes. The surface of the body is very cold. There may be diarrhoea of green water which spurts out. There is a metallic taste in the mouth. Face and skin may turn blue.

Areas of application Cholera. Colic. Convulsions. Cough. Diarrhoea. Teething. Whooping cough.

Pain Severe cramps.

Worse Touch. Hot weather. Overworking.

Better Stretching out (cramp). Cold drinks (vomiting and colic). Lying on stomach.

Copper

Drosera
Drosera rotundifolia
Sundew

This perennial carnivorous plant grows in the northern hemisphere. It likes wet conditions and closes its flower petals in strong sunlight, which is unusual in the plant kingdom. Insects are attracted to it, but once stuck, cannot escape, and

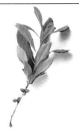
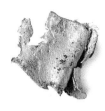
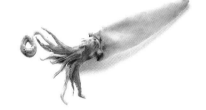

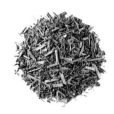

are dissolved by the plant's juices. Avoided by animals, it is known to cause coughing when eaten by sheep.

Characteristic symptoms
Predominantly a respiratory remedy, appropriate in cases of whooping cough, which manifests itself in deep barking fits which take the breath away, and may be accompanied by a nosebleed. During cough they hold their sides and may retch and vomit. There is a sensation in the throat like the tickling of a feather. They are much worse at night, as soon as their head touches the pillow.

Areas of application Asthma. Bronchitis. Measles. Whooping cough.

Worse After midnight. On lying down. After measles.

Better Pressure (holding the part relieves the pain in head and chest). Open air.

Dulcamara
Solanum dulcamara
Bittersweet, Woody nightshade

Found in England and Wales, woody nightshade enjoys a moist environment on woodland borders and in hedgerows. All parts of the plant are poisonous, including the red berries which appear in autumn. The remedy is made from the tender leaves and twigs.

Characteristic symptoms The major aggravation in this remedy is from

cold, damp weather or when the weather changes suddenly from hot to cold, as can be found on autumn days.

Areas of application Back pain. Complaints arising from moving in and out of an air-conditioned environment. Diarrhoea after a chill. Influenza. Rheumatism. Stiff neck. Summer colds. Tonsillitis. Whooping cough.

Pain Spasms of pain in the bowels.

Worse Sudden changes of temperature. Cold wet weather. Cold drinks and ice-creams. Autumn.

Better Warmth. Dry weather.

Echinacea
Echinacea angustifolia
Purple cone flower

This plant, which grows in the western United States, has a very powerful action on the blood and is considered a natural antibiotic. The remedy is made from a tincture of the whole fresh plant.

Purple cone flower

Characteristic symptoms Acts as a general blood cleanser. Use specifically for septic conditions caused by poisonous plants, or insect or animal bites, with offensive discharges. Tired, aching muscles with

weakness. Essential when travelling to areas where the water is unclean – add a few drops to all drinking water.

Areas of application Abscesses. After surgery. Blood poisoning. Boils. Carbuncles. Effects of vaccination. Gangrene. Poisonous bites (e.g. snake bites) and wounds. The pain of cancer. Typhoid.

Pain Tired, aching.

Worse Injury. Surgery. Cold air.

Better Lying. Rest.

Eupatorium Perf
Eupatorium perfoliatum
Boneset, Indian sage

Eupatorium perfoliatum grows in moist lowlands, swamps and on the banks of brooks and streams. Used by Native Americans in fevers, colds and bronchial disorders, it was considered a 'cure-all' because of its cleansing effect on almost all organs.

Characteristic symptoms Typical flu symptoms – very severe aching sore pains in muscles and bones; feel as if they are breaking. Intensely cold with shivers, or burning heat. Weakness, restlessness, nausea. Particularly helps the removal of catarrh.

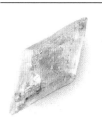
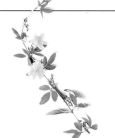

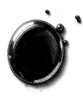
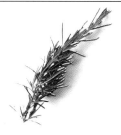

Areas of application Bone pains. Colds. Influenza.

Pain Violent aching, sore, bruised, as if bones are breaking.

Worse Cold air. Motion. Periodically.

Better Sweating. Talking. Vomiting bile.

Euphrasia
Euphrasia officinalis
Eyebright

As its name suggests, eyebright has consistently been used to strengthen eyes and treat eye disorders.

Eyebright

Characteristic symptoms Affects the mucous membranes of the eyes, nose and chest, producing catarrh and copious watery secretions. Eye secretions cause smarting of the skin, in contrast to a bland nasal discharge. This remedy is mainly used externally in the form of a tincture and can be taken internally if indicated.

Areas of application Conjunctivitis and eye disorders in measles. Eyestrain, especially when working with computers.

Pain Burning. Sore.

Worse Sunlight. Wind. Warmth.

Better Open air.

Ferrum Phos
Ferrum phosphoricum
White phosphate of iron

This biochemic tissue salt is prepared by mixing sodium phosphate and sulphate of iron. An oxygen carrier, it is part of the haemoglobin in the blood. It also has the capacity to strengthen the blood vessel walls, especially the arteries.

Characteristic symptoms Useful in the first stage of all acute illness where there is inflammation and fever. Symptoms to look for are pain, heat, swelling and redness. There is disturbed circulation and relaxation of tissue; haemorrhages are bright red. It can be used to stem the flow of blood from cuts by crushing a few pills and sprinkling the powder onto the injured part. Local congestions may give rise to throbbing headaches with earache, which are relieved by having a nosebleed.

Areas of application Anaemia. Colds. Coughs. Earache. Fever. Frostbite. Headache. Nosebleed. Minor haemorrhages.

Pain Throbbing. Burning rawness. Bruised. Sore.

Worse Heat of the sun. Motion.

Better Nosebleed. Cold applications.

Yellow jasmine

Gelsemium
Gelsemium sempervirens
Yellow jasmine

Yellow jasmine prefers woodland and coastal areas and is now a popular garden plant despite its poisonous properties.

Characteristic symptoms Overpowering heaviness, weakness and soreness. Drowsy, with heavy, drooping eyelids. Trembling. Chills and heat up and down the spine. Weakness remaining after flu. Weakness of the knees and unsteady while walking. Nervous excitement before important events leading to frequent emptying of the bladder, or diarrhoea. Symptoms brought on by shock or fright. Mental confusion including that resulting from drug treatment. Absence of thirst during fever.

Areas of application Fevers. Influenza. Measles. Teething babies. Drug intoxification. Shocks. Ordeals such as interviews, exams, public speaking.

Pain Tremendous aching and soreness of muscles.

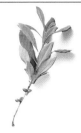
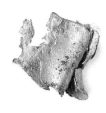
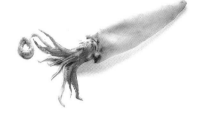

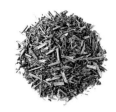

Worse Anticipation. Surprises. Humid weather. Heat of the sun. Cold, damp weather.

Better Profuse urination. Sweating.

Glonoine
Nitroglycerine

Also known as dynamite, which gives a clear indication of its area of use in homeopathic potency – symptoms are of an explosive, bursting, violent nature.

Characteristic symptoms Bursting, throbbing headaches as if head is expanding. Blood rushes upwards. Of great use in sunstroke. Headaches after monthly period suddenly stops, or is very heavy. Dizzy on standing up.

Areas of application Headaches. Neuralgia. Sunstroke. Vertigo.

Pain Throbbing. Bursting. Stabbing. Tearing. Pounding.

Worse Any form of heat to the head. Sun. The slightest jarring. Light.

Better Cold things.

Hamamelis
Hamamelis virginica
Witch hazel

This is a deciduous shrub which grows in Canada and the United States. Its habitat is damp woods and the banks of streams. It has yellow flowers in the autumn, and the seeds ripen the following year. Divining rods have traditionally been made from this shrub, which may be one reason for its popular name. It is used externally as a tincture as well as in homeopathic potency.

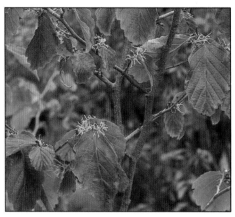

Witch hazel

Characteristic symptoms The main area of action of Hamamelis is the veins – of the rectum, genitals, limbs and throat. Piles and varicose veins in pregnancy and after childbirth. There is a full, bursting feeling in the veins. Apply externally to open, painful wounds and burns, and to varicosed areas. Relieves pain after operations. There may be minor haemorrhages of dark blood.

Areas of application After surgery. Burns. Cuts and abrasions. Nosebleeds. Piles. Varicose veins.

Pain Sore. Bruised. Prickling. Stinging. Cutting.

Worse Touch. Pressure. During the day.

Hepar Sulph
Hepar sulphuris calcareum
Sulphide of calcium

An impure sulphide of calcium made by burning the white interior of oyster shell with pure flowers of sulphur.

Characteristic symptoms An over-sensitive person who is aggravated by being 'touched' mentally or from physical touch of the painful part. Hard to please and can become very angry if disturbed. They are extremely sensitive to cold air. All discharges smell bad like rotting cheese. Wounds become septic with much pus. Tonsils and neck glands swell and throat pain travels to ears on swallowing. For croupy, barking coughs, where there is much rattling of loose phlegm which is difficult to bring up. Child cries before coughing. The cough is worse for cold drinks and any exposure to the slightest draught, such as putting the hands out of the bed covers. Helps bring splinters to the surface.

Areas of application Abscess. Athlete's foot. Catarrh. Cold sores. Croupy coughs. Earache. Glandular swellings. Mastitis. Quinsy. Splinters. Styes. Tonsillitis. Toothache.

Pain Like needles or splinters.

Worse Draughts. Uncovering. Touch. Lying on the painful part. Cold air and cold drinks.

Better Heat. Wrapping up warmly. Moist weather. Tobacco.

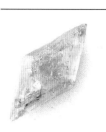
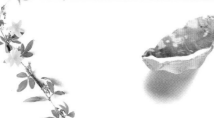
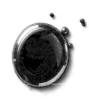
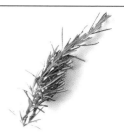

Hypericum

Hypericum perfoliatum
St John's wort

Found throughout the British Isles, it grows near road verges, hedgebanks, on grassland, meadows and open woodlands. Its small yellow flowers are accompanied by black-spotted leaves. When leaves are held up to the light, the spots look like holes but are glands containing blood-red oil. This plant was used in medieval times and was considered valuable in exorcising evil spirits – the name Hypericum is Greek for 'over an apparition'.

Characteristic symptoms Wherever nerves are injured, especially where the skin has been punctured by a rusty nail; or animal or insect bite. Injuries are more painful than they look. Helps with pain after surgery, a forceps delivery, dental work. Prevents tetanus if given immediately (see Tetanus, page 46). Unable to walk after accident to spine, especially where the coccyx is involved. After injuries where the person feels as if he had been lifted high up and has fear of falling. Pain in the stump after amputations.

Areas of application Amputations. Bites of insects and animals. Cuts. Damage to fingers and toes. Dental

treatment. Forceps delivery. Frostbite. Neuralgia. Painful scars. Puncture wounds. Spinal injuries, especially the coccyx. Surgery. Tetanus. Use also externally to bathe wounds.

Pain Violent shooting pain along nerve pathways. Burning, tingling, numbness.

Worse Shock. Touch.

Better Rubbing.

St John's wort

Ignatia

Ignatia amara
St Ignatia's bean

This tree grows in the Philippines. In the days of plague, people carried a bean believing it would work as a prophylactic against the disease. Homeopaths have used this remedy successfully to treat plague. Like Nux Vomica, the seeds contain strychnine, but symptom pictures of the two remedies are very different.

Characteristic symptoms The remedy is of particular use where there is shock resulting from the death of a relative or friend, stillbirth or separation from a relationship. There may be silent suffering with sighing or floods of uncontrollable tears. Symptoms change rapidly with contradictory effects. For example, the feeling of having a lump in the throat is not painful when swallowing solids

(unusual), but is worse when not swallowing. An empty, sinking feeling in the stomach is not improved by eating. There is toothache after coffee and smoking; pain which shoots up the rectum; a sensation of a lump in various parts. Profuse urination relieves some symptoms.

Areas of application Bereavement, separation. Depression. Fainting. Fear and anxiety. Miscarriage. Plague. Sadness. Shock. Sobbing. Sore throat.

Pain Spasms. Jerking and twitching. Nervous shuddering with pain.

Worse Shock. Anger. Worrying. Open air. Tobacco. Coffee. Touch.

Better Urination. Deep breath. Eating. Swallowing. Alone.

Ipecac

Cephaelis ipecacuanha
Ipecacuanha

This root has been used widely as an expectorant in cough medicines. It is a shrub which likes damp conditions and grows in parts of South America.

Characteristic symptoms The three main areas are gastric disturbances, respiratory problems and haemorrhages. Constant nausea is present with most symptoms, often with a clean, uncoated tongue (unusual). Vomiting does not relieve the nausea. Haemorrhage of bright red blood is accompanied by nausea. Stomach feels as if hanging down.

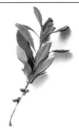
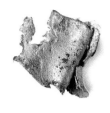

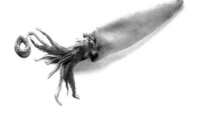
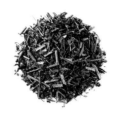

Aggravated by rich food, fruits, berries, raisins, sweets. Suffocating coughs from an accumulation of mucus. Child goes stiff with a bluish-red face and eventually vomits. Whooping cough with nosebleeds. Threatened miscarriage with cutting pain around the navel. Nausea precedes headaches. Hard to please.

Areas of application Asthma. Fainting from heat. Gastric flu. Haemorrhage. Miscarriage. Morning sickness. Nausea. Nosebleed. Pregnancy. Vomiting. Whooping cough.

Pain Bruised. Crushed. Cutting. Griping.

Worse Over-eating. Rich food. Warmth. Damp. Heat and cold. Vomiting. Over-eating. Tobacco.

Better Open air. Cold drinks. Rest.

Kali Bic
Kali bichromicum
Bichromate of potash

Bichromate of potash is manufactured from chrome iron ore and has been widely used in the arts for dyeing and printing, as woodstain, in photography and in electric batteries.

Bichromate of potash

Characteristic symptoms Mucous membranes of the air passages are affected. Pressure and a stuffed-up sensation at the root of the nose; the frontal sinuses are also blocked (worse in the warmth, better in the cool air). Violent sneezing, worse in the morning. Loss of smell. Pains in small spots which may change suddenly. Pain in throat or tongue on sticking the tongue out. Sensation as if hair on tongue or in nostril. Bones of face feel bruised. Discharges are stringy, tough, thick and greenish-yellow.

Areas of application Catarrh. Headaches. Blocked, painful sinuses.

Pain Sharp, stitching.

Worse Cold. Damp. Morning. Summer heat. Beer (indigestion).

Better Heat. Motion. Pressure.

Kali Carb
Kali carbonicum
Potassium carbonate

Potassium carbonate originated through the needs of commerce, particularly in the soap and glass-making industries. It was extracted from the ashes of wood and plants.

Characteristic symptoms Weakness runs throughout this remedy. Back feels broken (better

lying down). Backache after childbirth. Debilitating states after miscarriage and labour. As if back or legs will give out while walking. Sudden sharp pains up or down the back extending down the thighs to the knees, or pain travels from hip to knee. Baggy swelling around the eyes, especially the upper lid. Easy sweating. Catches cold easily. Yawns a lot. An irritable person. Asthma, worse for the least movement, better bending head forwards.

Areas of application Asthma. Backache. Labour. Weakness.

Pain Sharp stitching. Stabbing. Burning. Throbbing. Numbness and coldness.

Worse Cold. Touch. Night. Lying on painful side.

Better Warmth. Open air. Bent forwards with elbows on knees.

Kali Mur
Kali muriaticum
Potassium chloride

Potassium chloride is found in nature as a mineral called carnallite. It is a constituent of blood corpuscles, nerve and brain cells, muscles and inter-cellular fluids.

Characteristic symptoms Useful for all sluggish conditions. A deficiency of this tissue salt gives rise to thick, white discharges and the blood thickens. There is chronic catarrh of the middle ear leading to deafness.

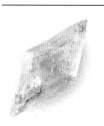
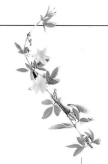
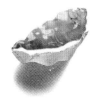
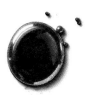
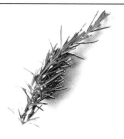

Noises in the ear on blowing the nose or swallowing. Stuffy head colds. Glandular swellings, especially around the ears. Whiteness of tongue. In babies with thrush, the mucous membranes of the mouth are milky white and blistered. Indigestion from fatty or rich foods. Pale-coloured stools with soreness around the anus.

Areas of application: Acne. Catarrh. Colds. Constipation. Cradle cap. Dandruff. Earache. Indigestion. Jet travel. Mouth ulcers (canker sores). Thrush (yeast). Tonsillitis.

Pain Sore.

Worse Fatty foods. Rich food. Open air.

Better Cold drinks.

Kali Phos
Kali phosphoricum
Potassium phosphate

Kali Phos is found in all fluids and tissues of the body, particularly the nerves, brain, blood cells and muscles. It acts as an antiseptic and delays the decay of tissues.

Characteristic symptoms Symptoms that come on from slight causes. Can be used where there is over-sensitivity, exhaustion from worrying, nervousness and anxiety, all leading to sleeplessness. Kali Phos soothes and calms an overspent nervous system. Headache from mental strain while studying or overworking. Bad memory

for names or words. Palpitations from over-excitement. Pains with sensation of paralysis. Noise startles easily. Sweats after the least effort. Useful where weakness remains after influenza.

Areas of application: Asthma. Poor concentration. Excitement. Fear and anxiety. Jet travel. Neuralgia. Palpitations. Sleeplessness.

Pain Stitching. Sharp stinging. Aching.

Worse Worrying. Excitement. Mental and physical exertion. Cold.

Better Heat. Sleep. Eating.

Kali Sulph
Kali sulphuricum
Potassium sulphate

This substance occurs naturally in volcanic lava. Combined with Ferrum Phos, it is an oxygen carrier. A deficiency causes yellowy-green discharges.

Characteristic symptoms Yellowy-green discharges – thin, watery, sticky. Yellow dandruff, yellow slimy tongue, yellow vaginal discharge (leucorrhoea). Scaly eruptions of the skin. Loss of taste and smell with catarrh.

Areas of application: Asthma. Catarrh. Colds. Coughs with rattling chest. Conjunctivitis. Dandruff. Earache. Rheumatism (worse from heat).

Pain Stitching. Tearing.

Worse Warmth. Stuffy room. Evening.

Better Cool. Open air.

Lachesis
Trigonocephalus lachesis
Bushmaster, Surukuku snake

The symptoms of this remedy were originally obtained by Constantine Hering, a homeopath who travelled to the Amazon in 1827 to collect plant

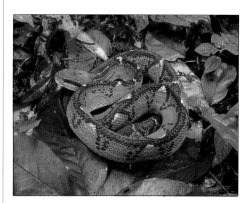

Bushmaster snake

and animal specimens for the German government. The story is told of how he offered a reward for a live specimen of the bushmaster or surukuku snake. As soon as it was delivered, in a bamboo box, everyone fled in terror – everyone except Hering. As he handled the snake, although not bitten, he was affected by the fumes of the powerful venom and became delirious. During this poisoning, his wife noted all his symptoms. From that time, he was unable to wear a collar because he could not tolerate restriction around his throat, an important symptom of the remedy.

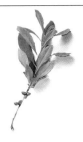 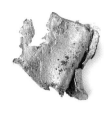 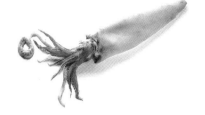 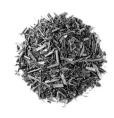

Characteristic symptoms The left side of the body is mainly affected but symptoms may move from the left to the right. There is a sensation of a lump anywhere, particularly in the throat and abdomen. There is a feeling of constriction – in throat, head, or anus. During a sore throat, much pain is experienced swallowing saliva (empty swallowing), but there is no difficulty with swallowing solids. There is excessive sensitivity of the skin. A sense of suffocation on falling asleep. Better for the onset of a discharge, e.g. in days leading up to the menses there may be great irritability and tension, which is immediately relieved as soon as the blood starts to flow; or a headache will feel better for the release of nasal catarrh. Septic states with blueness or mottling of the affected part.

People who need this remedy may say they feel full of poison; they are frequently lively and talkative, and in conversation they will change subject rapidly. There may be a history of jealousy and vindictiveness in their character.

Areas of application: Bites of poisonous animals. Boils. Carbuncles. Frostbite. Gangrene. Headaches. Before menstruation. Mumps. Nosebleeds (instead of menses). Quinsy. Sore throats.

Pain Throbbing, pulsing like a hammer.

Worse On falling asleep. After sleep. The slightest touch. Pressure of clothes. Cloudy weather. Spring, summer. Heat of the sun. Empty swallowing. Hot drinks. Suppressed discharges.

Better Swallowing solids. Cold drinks. Cool, open air.

Ledum
Ledum palustre
Wild rosemary

Wild rosemary grows in damp, marshy regions of northern Europe. It is largely avoided by grazing animals with the exception of goats, which will eat it. Its properties have led to wild rosemary being used for a variety of purposes, including keeping lice off pigs and oxen, preventing flour from going mouldy and in beer to increase its intoxicating effects. It is also used as an expectorant in cough medicines.

Characteristic symptoms The person feels intensely cold, as does the injured part, though it is relieved by cold application. This remedy has a special action on the capillaries and is therefore of use for a bloodshot, bruised or black eye after a blow (for pain in the eyeball, *see* Symphytum). Parts become blue, purple and puffy. There is weakness, numbness or twitching of the part. The effects of old injuries. Puncture wounds, for instance, from rusty nails or insect stings. Used in conjunction with Hypericum, it can prevent tetanus.

Areas of application: Abscess. Bites and stings. Boils. Bone injuries. Bruises. Carbuncles. Eye injuries. Puncture wounds. Septic conditions. Sprains. Tetanus.

Pain Throbbing. Tearing. Pricking. Shoots upward. Stiff. Sore.

Worse Warmth.

Better Cold; cold bathing.

Lycopodium
Lycopodium clavatum
Clubmoss, Wolf's claw

The habitat of this plant is hilly pastures and heaths in central and northern Europe, Russia and North America, and it is especially common in the north of Britain. Fossilized remains of this moss have been found, which indicate that at one time it had a prominent place in the world's vegetation.

The remedy is made from a tincture of the spores. Clubmoss has been used to produce stage lightning at theatres, pharmaceutically as a dusting powder to coat pills to prevent them from sticking to each other, and by herbalists in skin disorders and kidney complaints. Mostly, it has been considered to be an inert substance, but its use in homeopathy has shown otherwise.

Characteristic symptoms Complaints appear on the right side or go from the right to the left (the opposite of Lachesis). Mental strength with physical weakness typifies this remedy. Often an intellectual type –

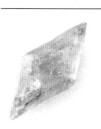
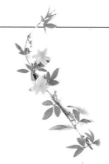
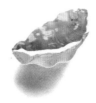
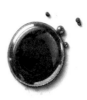
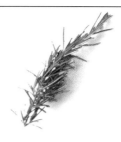

in children, manifesting itself as a bookworm rather than an interest in physical sports. An irritable, fussy, flatulent person. Indecisive. Timid. Lacks confidence and has anxiety in the abdomen before undertaking something new. Has a strong affinity with the digestive area – eating very small amounts fills them up quickly. Missing a meal may cause a headache and in the abdomen there is much rumbling and flatulence, especially after eating wind-inducing foods such as cabbage and beans. Hunger in the night. Desire for sweet foods. Must take food and drink while it is still very hot. Constipation when travelling or when away from home. Much irritability and anger arising from upset liver. Oversensitive to pain, which suddenly comes and goes. Prefers fresh air but gets cold.

Areas of application: Constipation. Loss of confidence. Indigestion. Flatulence. Irritability. Right-sided ear and throat symptoms. Mouth-breathing from blocked nose and sinuses. Wakeful at night. Sexual exhaustion.

Pain Raw. Burning.

Worse On waking in the morning and from 4–8 p.m. Eating, even very small amounts. Pressure of clothes. Cold drinks and food. Milk. Vegetables, beans, bread and pastry.

Better Hot food and drinks. Passing gas.

Mag Phos
Magnesium phosphoricum
Magnesium phosphate

Known as the anti-spasmodic tissue salt, the main area of action with Mag Phos is on the nervous system and muscles. It is an important constituent of brain, bone, nerves, muscles, blood and sperm. Deficiencies cause spasms, paralysis and cramps. It is made from magnesium sulphate and sodium phosphate, which form into six-sided, needle-like crystals. It is found in beer and cereal grains.

Characteristic symptoms This remedy brings great relief from many types of spasmodic pain. Sudden violent pains which shoot like lightning, causing the person to bend double. Muscular twitchings. Pains rapidly change place. Cries out with pain. Stomach cramps. Menstrual cramps which are relieved by the flow. Babies with colic. Complaints brought on by standing in cold water. This remedy will act faster if dissolved in warm water and slowly sipped.

Areas of application: Asthma. Backache. Colic. Diarrhoea. Earache. Headaches. Hiccoughs. Menstrual pain. Neuralgia. Sciatica. Spasmodic cough. Teething. Toothache. Whooping cough. Writer's/musician's cramp.

Pain Shooting. Darting. Stabbing. Spasmodic cramps. All types of pain except burning.

Worse Washing, swimming or standing in cold water. Cold air. Touch. Night.

Better Warmth. Hot bath. Rest. Bending double. Pressure.

Merc Sol
Mercurius solubilis
Mercury, Quicksilver

Mercury *Made from soluble black oxide of mercury precipitated from a solution in nitric acid by using caustic ammonia, Merc Sol was conceived by Samuel Hahnemann and substituted for the corrosive mercurial salts which were at that time popular with physicians. Many acute and chronic poisonings have arisen from the use of mercury. It has been used extensively in medicine, especially to treat syphilis and as a purgative; in commerce in the making of felt hats ('mad as a hatter' and 'hatter's shakes' are picturesque references to its effects on the nervous system), to make mirrors, thermometers and barometers, and as a dusting powder for fingerprinting. Its use continues in fungicides, herbicides, some water-based paints and in dentistry for amalgam fillings.*

Characteristic symptoms The people who respond well to this remedy are

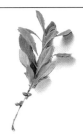
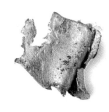

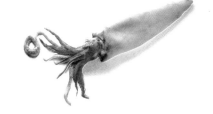
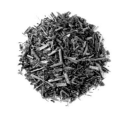

'mercurial' in nature – quick and fluid in their movements, like the quicksilver in a barometer which is influenced by the slightest change in temperature. They are changeable and uncertain, speak very fast or may stammer. There is weakness and trembling of limbs or tongue. Offensiveness of breath and sweat; bodily discharges which may burn and be greenish-yellow. There is often a metallic taste in the mouth, an increased flow of saliva and bleeding gums. Ulcerated mouth, throat, tonsils or genitals. Throat pain travels to the ears on swallowing. Glandular swellings. Very easily overheated or chilled – like a human barometer. They catch cold easily and colds often travel upwards, e.g. to the eyes. Drenching night sweats.

Areas of application: Abscess. Bleeding gums. Earache with discharge. Joint pain. Mumps. Rheumatism. Shingles. Sore throat. Quinsy. Teething (with increased flow of saliva). Tonsillitis.

Pain Burning. Raw. Sore. Pricking like needles. Stinging (like Apis).

Worse Night. Heat. Cold. Weather changes. Sweating. Draughts. Heat of bed. Lying on right side. During and after urination. Touching cold objects.

Better Rest.

Mezereum
Daphne mezereum
Spurge olive

This hardy shrub found growing in hilly woodlands on chalk or limestone in Europe, Siberia and North America is now very rare in England, having been heavily gathered for domestic cultivation. It flowers from February to April before the leaves appear. Although the berries are poisonous and have caused death in children, the bark has been used to alleviate symptoms after snake bites. Redness and blistering appear on skin which is rubbed with the leaves or bark. The remedy is made from fresh bark collected just before the plant flowers.

Spurge olive

Characteristic symptoms Neuralgia of teeth and face after shingles. Internal burning with violent itching externally. The itching is unbearable, worse for warmth and changes place on scratching. Face pain may be relieved by radiated heat from a fire. Pains radiate and shoot downwards and are followed by chilliness and numbness. One-sided symptoms.

Areas of application: Neuralgia after shingles. Decayed teeth roots.

Pain Violent burning, like fire. Radiating. Shooting.

Worse The slightest cold air. Warmth of bed. Night. Touch. Warm bath. Suppressed eczema.

Better Wrapping up. Heat of a fire (face pain).

Nat Mur
Natrum muriaticum
Sodium chloride, Common salt

The free flow of water in the oceans is dependent upon the presence of salt, without which they would ice up. Likewise, in the human body, the movement of fluids between each cell is maintained by this essential mineral. Because of its water-attracting property, salt eaten in excessive amounts leads to water imbalance, and poisonous conditions may result. Overdosing can cause dryness of the skin, lips and mucous membranes, cracked lips, cold sores, bloatedness, increased sweating, headaches, depression and anaemia. On the other hand, the body may need salt where there is excessive sweating, for example, in hot weather, which can lead to tiredness and cramps (see Sunstroke).

Characteristic symptoms People who require Nat Mur are often thin, thirsty, tired, have cold feet and hands, and usually either crave salt or dislike it. They may feel tearful but have great difficulty letting the tears flow, preferring to be alone because sympathy makes them feel worse. Easily offended, they hold on to perceived slights and become resentful; this may continue for years.

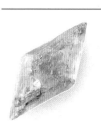
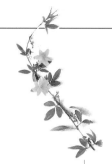
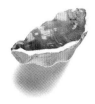
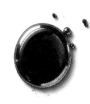
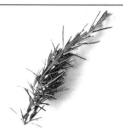

Easily depressed with a negative outlook. Tend to feel worse from sunrise to sunset. Excessive moisture or dryness are indications for this remedy. Frequently catches colds which have a watery or thick, white nasal discharge. Nose may drip like a tap or gets blocked high up. Loss of smell or taste with colds. Sneezing in the morning. Mucus tastes salty. Very thirsty for water. Cracks in middle of lower lip. Blistery spots. Constipation of dry, crumbly stools, worse at the seaside. Sneezing, coughing or laughing causes eyes to water.

Areas of Application
Anaemia. Catarrh. Cold sores. Colds. Constipation. Cracked lips, skin. Jet travel (swollen hands and feet). Mouth ulcers (canker sores). Pregnancy and labour. Sadness. Sunstroke. Suppressed tears. Water retention. Head injury.

Pain Throbbing, like hammers.

Worse For fuss or being comforted. Sunrise to sunset. Heat of the sun or room. Seaside. Storms. Full moon. 9 a.m. to 11 a.m. Alternate days.

Better Being alone. Open air. Eating snacks rather than full meals.

Nat Phos
Natrum phosphoricum
Sodium phosphate

Phosphoric acid and sodium carbonate are combined to give us sodium phosphate. This is used commercially to make such things as baking powder, detergents and photographic chemicals. It neutralizes acids in the blood and helps with the digestion of fats. When there is a deficiency, uric acid forms salts which settle in the joints, leading to stiffness and swelling.

Characteristic symptoms Acidity and sourness. Sour-smelling babies who may have been receiving large quantities of milk and sugar. Children grind teeth in sleep. Greenish diarrhoea. Deep, yellow, creamy discharges. Golden-yellow coating at back of tongue or tonsils. Children pick their nose and scratch their bottom (worms).

Rock salt

Areas of application Acidity. Gout. Indigestion. Joint pain. Morning sickness. Rheumatism. Worms.

Pain Pricking.

Worse Fat food. Sugar. Milk. Storms.

Better Cold.

Nat Sulph
Natrum sulphuricum
Sodium sulphate

Found in sea water, mineral spas and salt lakes, Nat Sulph can be bought in some places for laxative purposes under the name of Glauber Salts. It has an affinity with the head, liver and pancreas. It attracts water, like Nat Mur, but is concerned with eliminating any surplus from the body. Nat Mur distributes water and Nat Phos absorbs.

Characteristic symptoms Extreme sensitivity to anything damp and wet (damp houses, watery food, swimming, humid weather). Helpful during oppressive, humid weather to overcome lethargy. Mental troubles and headaches which come on after head injuries. Eyes sensitive to light. Hip joint pain on standing up or on getting out of bed in the morning. Inflammation around nail roots. A sense of fullness. Flatulent rumbling, gurgling bowels followed by noisy, spluttering stools (Arg Nit). Thick yellow-green pus or watery yellow blisters.

Areas of application Diarrhoea. Exhaustion from humid weather. Flatulent bloating. Hangnails. Head injuries. Joint pain. Sciatica.

Pain Piercing, throbbing, sharp, cutting.

Worse Damp, wet weather. Hot, humid weather. Warm room. Touch. Vegetables. Fruit. Starchy food. Late evening or morning. Lying on left side.

Better Open air. Warm, dry air. After breakfast.

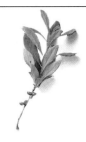
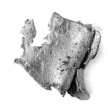

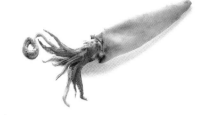
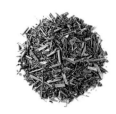

Nit Ac

Nitricum acidum

Nitric acid

This is a highly corrosive acid which burns the skin and turns it yellow. The fumes, which occur when Nit Ac comes into contact with moist air, can cause suffocation and death. It is used mainly in the manufacture of explosives and fertilizers as well as in lacquers, plastics, drugs and dyes.

Characteristic symptoms Anxiety about health. Tremble with anger or extremely irritable. Hateful to others. Very sensitive to noise, touch, pain, to any slight cause. Suffer a great deal if they lose sleep. Desires fatty foods, salt. A chilly person. The remedy acts strongly where there are symptoms affecting the outlets of the body – where mucuous membranes come to the surface – mouth, lips, nostrils, anus, genitals. Discharges are offensive and burn the parts they touch. Urine smells very strong, like that of a horse. Ulcerations, especially of the tonsils. There is a sharp splinter pain in the throat which goes to the ear on swallowing. Sharp pain while emptying bowels, which may continue for hours afterwards. Feels as if anus is torn. Very painful, bleeding piles. Useful for haemorrhage after piles operation.

Areas of application Earache. Piles. Bleeding. Ulcerated throat. Thrush (yeast). Tonsillitis.

Pain Splinter, like fishbone or glass, which is aggravated by movement or touching the area. Soreness.

Worse Loss of sleep. Touch. Noise. Cold, damp. Night. Milk and fats.

Better Riding in cars, etc.

Nux Vomica

Strychnos nux vomica

Poison nut

Strychnos nux vomica is a small evergreen tree which grows in Asia and northern Australia. After flowering it produces an orange-coloured fruit the size of an apple. Strychnine, a powerful stimulus to the central nervous system, is found in the bitter-tasting seeds, along with copper. The bitter wood of the tree has been used in India to treat snake bites and intermittent fever, and the leaves used externally in rheumatism.

Poisonings include increased sensitivity to noise, light and touch; spasms with extreme stiffness and rigidity of the whole body; a severe rise in blood pressure – leading to its administration in cases of surgical shock and cardiac failure – and convulsions, causing death by asphyxiation when the respiratory system fails.

Characteristic symptoms This remedy is very tranquilizing for people who are over-sensitive to all external stimuli. They are nervy, excitable, angry, impatient, irritable and continually nag and find fault in others. They may be worn out from overwork or neglect their body by indulging in too much coffee, alcohol, cigarettes, drugs or rich food. This leads to frequent digestive upsets and difficulty sleeping. There is a bitter, bad taste in mouth. Food causes pressure like a stone in the stomach, which is worse 2 or 3 hours after eating. Much difficulty is experienced in vomiting or opening the bowels, even though there is a constant urge – 'wants to but cannot'. Breastfed babies develop colic when the mother over-indulges in rich, spicy food or alcohol. Nosebleed or severe abdominal pain after piles operation. With a cold, nose may be blocked on one side while the other runs; nose is stuffed up at night, runs indoors. One nostril may be blocked while the other runs. Thoughts prevent sleep, or person wakes at 3 a.m. and is unable to return to sleep. Great desire for stimulants, which may be maintaining causes of unrest.

Areas of application Asthma. Colds. Coughs. Constipation. Fainting. Hangovers. Headache. Indigestion. Irritability. Labour. Menses, painful with urging to open bowels. Morning sickness. Nausea and vomiting. Nosebleed. Palpitations. Piles. Sleep loss. Vertigo.

Pain Raw. Sore. Bruised. Sticking.

Worse Morning. Cold, dry air, especially draughts. Loss of sleep. Touch. Noise. Light. Over-eating. Pepper. Coffee. Alcohol. Drugs. Purgatives. Tight clothes around waist.

Better Resting. Moist air. Hot drinks. Milk. Fats.

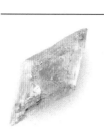
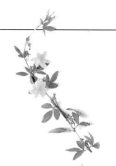

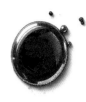
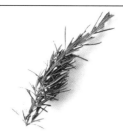

Petroleum
Oleum petrae
Crude rock oil

People working in the petroleum industry are prone to a variety of complaints including skin diseases, anaemia, dyspepsia, insomnia and irritability. The remedy is made from purified commercial petroleum. For first aid purposes, it is used for travel sickness and sickness in pregnancy.

Characteristic symptoms Nausea and vomiting brought on by motion of boats, cars, etc. Feels worse in the open air (which is the opposite to Tabacum, which is better outdoors). Nausea when hungry; after eating; with headaches; in the morning, especially in pregnancy; mouth fills with water. Stomach feels weak and empty. Extremely hungry in the night, or after emptying bowels. Back of head feels heavy. Dizzy on standing up.

Areas of application Morning sickness of pregnancy. Nausea and vomiting. Travel sickness.

Worse Motion of boats or cars. Open air. Eating. Morning. Pregnancy. Lying with head low.

Better Warm air. Lying with head high.

Phosphorus
The element

This non-metallic element is an important constituent of animal and plant life. In the human body, it is found mostly in bones and the insulating covering of nerve sheaths, brain and spinal cord. In its yellow form, it is a highly dangerous poison. Phosphorus fumes in chemical and match factories have poisoned many people working with it and one of the diseases it gave rise to was known as 'phossy jaw' – a condition where the lower jaw gradually disintegrated and sound teeth fell out. Nowadays red phosphorus, which is much less harmful, is used to make matches and fertilizers. Because it ignites as soon as it is in contact with air, it is stored under water. The name Phosphorus means 'light-bearer' and the remedy is frequently given to gregarious, out-going people who are the 'life and soul of the party'.

Characteristic symptoms Often required by tall people and children who grow very fast. Restless, nervous and look delicate. They love company and to be comforted; because of this, children will not want to go to bed alone and they are also afraid of the dark. There is great sensitivity to noise (they jump suddenly), smells, light, touch. Symptoms come and go suddenly. They bleed easily and small wounds bleed a lot. May have a sudden haemorrhage during an operation or an episiotomy in childbirth; a nosebleed instead of a period. There is burning or heat, particularly in the face, chest and up the spine. Burning thirst for cold or ice-cold drinks, which may be vomited after becoming warm in the stomach. Empty, hollow feeling in the chest or stomach. Hunger soon after a meal or ravenously hungry in the night. Must eat often or feels faint. With chest complaints, unable to lie on the left side, or the painful side. Colds settle on the chest. Crave salt, ice-cream, chocolate.

Areas of application Bronchitis. Descending colds. Coughs. Fainting. Fever. Haemorrhage. Hoarseness. Nausea and vomiting. Nosebleed. Surgery.

Pain Burning. Stitching.

Worse Lying on left side or painful side. Cold. Twilight. Sudden weather changes. Thunderstorms. Sight of water. Talking (cough). Being alone. Dark.

Better Eating. Sleep. Cold drinks and food. Lying on right side.

Phytolacca
Phytolacca decandra
Poke root

Phytolacca decandra is a perennial plant with a very thick root, sometimes as thick as a man's leg. It prefers a damp habitat and is found as far afield as China, North

Poke root

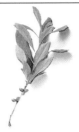
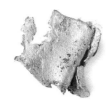
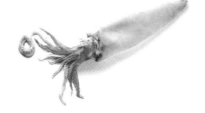

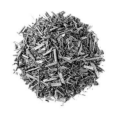

America, North Africa and Mediterranean countries. Although many poisonings have been recorded as a result of eating the plant's berries, drinking the tincture, or inhaling dust from the powdered dried root, it has a reputation in herbal medicine for the treatment of rheumatism, cancerous tumours, and helps cows with lactating difficulties such as mastitis.

Meadow anemone

Characteristic symptoms The glands, muscles and joints are particularly affected. Stony-hard swellings, stiff neck and body aches all over. Abscess of breastfeeding with fever and restlessness – breasts heavy and tender; pain while nursing, which spreads outwards. Nipples extremely sensitive and cracked. In mumps, glands at the angle of the jaws are swollen. In tonsillitis, dark red throat, unable to swallow hot drinks. Pain goes to both ears on swallowing, with pain at the root of the tongue. In teething, babies bite their gums together very hard.

Areas of application Breastfeeding. Earache. Mumps. Teething. Tonsillitis.

Pain Sore. Aching. Burning. Radiates outwards. Comes and goes suddenly.

Worse Swallowing hot drinks.

Better Biting something hard. Pressure (holds breasts).

Pulsatilla
Pulsatilla nigricans
Meadow anemone, Pasque flower, Wind flower

The meadow anemone has a liking for sunny pastures on well-drained soil, and is often found growing at the edge of woods or on hillsides in central and northern Europe and southern England. It has deep purple flowers in spring and autumn. Legend has it that the plant sprang from the tears of Venus and the remedy, which is made from the entire plant when in flower, is well known among homeopaths for its easy ability to cry.

Characteristic symptoms
Affectionate, timid, mild-natured. Can also be jealous and self-centred. Great changeability of moods and symptoms. Very touchy and cries at the slightest opportunity. Women cry when they are breastfeeding. Love sympathy and company. Children cling, whine and won't stay alone. Chilly people, but dislike heat and stuffy rooms, preferring the open air. Heaviness anywhere. Stomach feels as if it has a stone in it. Thirstlessness – dry mouth without thirst. Catarrhal states – eyes, ears, nose – discharges are thick, yellow or yellowy-green, bland (don't sting or create soreness). Useful in earache where a discharge has disappeared after antibiotics. Coughs dry at night, loose in the morning. Shortness of breath and weight on chest. Must sit up to cough. Mumps which travel to breasts or testicles. In fevers they are chilly, worse for warmth, and thirstless. Veins feel full. Anaemia from over-use of iron pills.

Areas of application Asthma. Breastfeeding. Bronchitis. Catarrh. Chickenpox. Chilblains. Conjunctivitis. Diarrhoea. Earache. Fever. Headaches. Indigestion. Labour. Measles. Miscarriage. Morning sickness. Mumps. Nausea and vomiting. Nosebleed. Styes. Tearfulness. Throat. Thrush (yeast). Toothache. Varicose veins. Vertigo.

Pain Changeable.

Worse Warm stuffy room. Rich, fatty food. Pork. Long after eating. Lying with head low. Getting feet wet. Wet, windy weather. Evening.

Better Cool open air. Walking gently in fresh air. Cold drinks and food. Lying with head high or sitting up. After a good cry.

Pyrogen
Pyrogenium
Sepsin

This remedy is made by leaving a piece of lean beef to decompose in the sun for 2 or 3 weeks, then potentizing it in the usual way! Its chief areas of homoeopathic use have been in typhoid fevers and blood poisoning.

 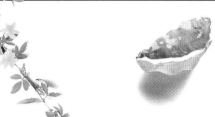 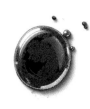 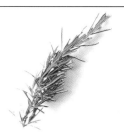

Characteristic symptoms Septic states with aching all over, soreness and exhaustion. Bone pains. Chronic complaints that date back to a septic condition (for example after surgery), typhoid fever or infection as a result of childbirth. All discharges are very smelly and offensive – sweat, vomit, menses, stools. Talks very fast. In fever, a sense of having several arms and legs, or of duality, feels like two different people.

Areas of application Abortion. Abscess. Any lingering septic condition. Boils. Blood poisoning. Fever after childbirth. Miscarriage. After surgery. Typhoid.

Pain Aching. Bruised. Sore. Burning.

Worse Cold. Damp. Moving eyes.

Better Heat. Hot bath. Changing position. Walking.

Rhus Tox
Rhus toxicondendron
Poison ivy

Poison ivy is found growing in North America. The remedy is made from a tincture of fresh leaves gathered at sunset just before the plant flowers. People are commonly poisoned by being in the vicinity of this plant especially after sunset, in damp weather. It causes itching, blistering and inflammation of the skin.

Characteristic symptoms Unable to relax in any position; stiffens up

during rest. Worse for initial movement, better once gets started. Tongue may have triangular red tip.

Areas of application Abscesses, boils, especially in armpit after delivery. Blood poisoning. Carbuncles. Hot, painful swelling of joints. Nettlerash. Rheumatism. Severe uterine pain after long delivery. Shingles. Sprains and injuries to fibrous tissue, ligaments and joints. Threatened abortion from straining, over-stretching.

Pain Burning, tearing, shooting, stitching. Bruised, sore, stiff.

Worse Night. Cold, wet weather. Before storms; change of weather. Getting chilled or wet after being hot. Ice-cream or ice-cold drinks on a hot day. Over-exertion, over-lifting. Initial movement.

Better Heat. Very hot baths. Movement. Walking in fresh air.

Ruta
Ruta graveolens
Rue

Rue

The remedy is made from the whole fresh plant of the common Rue, which grows in southern Europe. In the past it was used as a protection to keep plague at bay.

Characteristic symptoms Aching with restlessness. Intense weariness. Similar in its field of action to Rhus

Tox. Bone injuries, especially to the covering of the bone (periosteum). Hamstrings feel shortened. Thighs feel broken.

Areas of application Injuries to bones, tendons, cartilage, periosteum; joints, especially wrists, fingers. Lameness. Pain in the bones of the feet and ankles. Prolapse of rectum after giving birth. Sciatica. Sprains, strains. Useful for those working with computers – eyestrain, overuse of hands. Bone pain after dental work.

Pain Gnawing, digging, burning. Bruised, sore, as if beaten. Bones as if broken. Pain deep in bones. Cramp (in tongue).

Worse Over-exertion. Lying: parts lain on become sore. Touch. Cold, wet weather.

Better Lying on back (with backache). Warmth.

Secale
Secale cornutum
Ergot of rye

Ergot is the black, horn-shaped spur of the fungus Claviceps purpurea, which chooses rye grains as its home base. Ergot causes prolonged contractions of certain muscle fibres, especially those of the womb. For this reason it has been used in childbirth for several hundred years. Large epidemics of poisoning occurred in

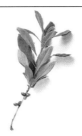
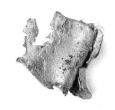

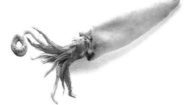
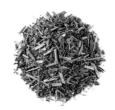

the Middle Ages in Germany and France – and more recently in Ethiopia – among people who ate bread made from rye diseased by this fungus. The poisonings were known as 'Ergotism', or St Anthony's Fire, and brought on hallucinations, spasmodic muscular contractions, severe pain with the gradual onset of gangrene in fingers and toes. Convulsions and haemorrhages led to death. Cows fed on infected grass lost their calves early. The remedy is made from a tincture of fresh spurs collected just before the rye is harvested.

Cuttlefish

Characteristic symptoms
Burning like fire in body; external parts are icy-cold, yet they refuse to be covered up. Cold clammy sweat. Threatened abortion at third month. Prolonged bearing down pains or no expulsive power in labour. As if everything is loose and open. After-pains too long and excessive. Prolapse of womb after forceps delivery. Septic placenta. Dark, offensive green lochia (the discharge after childbirth). Have never fully recovered since having an abortion or miscarriage. Tingling, numbness, stiffness and a crawling sensation. Big thirst for sour things, or lemonade.

Areas of application Abortion. Miscarriage. Childbirth. Blood poisoning. Gangrene. Septic placenta.

Pain Burning like fire. Cramps. Sharp. Stinging. Pricking.

Worse Warmth. Being covered. Touch. Labour. After abortion or forceps delivery.

Better Being fanned. Uncovering. Cold and cold bathing.

Sepia
Sepia officinalis
Cuttlefish, Squid

The remedy is made from a liquid contained in the inkbag of the cuttlefish. The liquid was known as Indian ink and widely used by artists. Squid prefer to swim on their own and will create a smoke-screen of brownish ink around themselves if they sense danger.

Characteristic symptoms The person needing this remedy tends to feel sluggish and sags mentally and bodily, but their energy increases if they do vigorous exercise such as aerobics. They feel over-burdened and are very irritable, may 'switch off' and become indifferent to their surroundings and people they love. Very easily offended.

Areas of application Backache. Constipation. Cystitis. Fainting. Hot flushes at menopause. Incontinence. Insomnia. Miscarriage. Morning sickness in pregnancy. Painful periods, PMT. Prolapse of womb. Thrush (yeast). Toothache.

Pain Dragging down in pelvis, aching especially of the lower back. Burning, shooting, pains in cervix or vagina.

Worse From being contradicted, comforted, noise, smells, touch. Going hungry. Boiled milk. Pregnancy. Before menses. Cold, windy weather. Snow.

Better Eating. Sleep. Crossing legs (womb pain). Strenuous exercise such as a fast walk, dancing, aerobics.

Silica
Silica terra
Pure flint

Silica is a major constituent of the earth's crust and sea sand. In its pure crystallized form it is rock crystal, quartz or flint. It does not occur freely in nature but has to be separated by chemical means. Plants depend on it for their ability to stand up straight. It is found in the human body in nerve sheaths, bone, periosteum (bone covering) and skin and imparts a sheen to hair and nails. Thinking is said to be improved if there is a plentiful supply in the connective tissue of the brain. The glass-making industry uses silica to give hardness and stability to its products.

Characteristic symptoms A chilly, timid but obstinate personality. Anticipates will fail in their normal business, from loss of confidence, but very capable once they begin, e.g. speaking in public. Lack of action or 'grit', seen in slow maturing of boils, styes, etc, which may harden instead of coming to a head. Sensitive to draughts, cold, noise. Every little injury goes septic and refuses to heal. Offensive, thick yellow discharges.

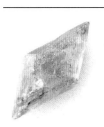
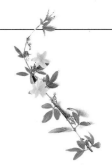
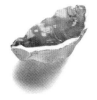

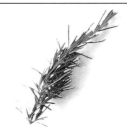

Smelly feet. Symptoms from suppressed foot sweat. Sweats on head. Helps bring splinters to the surface. Colds with earache. Colds go to chest. Coughs up smelly lumps of phlegm.

Areas of application Abscesses. Acne. Bedwetting. Boils. Colds. Coughs. Constipation (stool slips back in). Earache. Eye inflammation. Swollen glands. Hair and nails split. Injuries and neglected injuries. Septic wounds. Sinusitis. Splinters. Styes. Tonsillitis. Ulcerated throat. Ill effects of vaccination.

Pain Violent, sharp, shooting, pricking.

Flint

Worse Combing hair. Draughts. Open air. Touch. Before and during storms. Full moon. Cold drinks.

Better Wrapping up warmly, especially head. Warm room.

CAUTION: Because of its centrifugal action, Silica has the ability to move things to the surface, and should not be given if foreign bodies are lodged next to vital organs, or where there has been tuberculosis.

Spongia
Spongia tosta
Roasted sea sponge

This was originally classified as a plant but later found to have more in common with the animal kingdom. Roasting the sponge partially liberates its iodine. According to Hahnemann, toasted sponge was first referred to in the 13th century for use in goitre.

Characteristic symptoms Give after Aconite in croup when Aconite is no longer helping. Great dryness of the mucous membranes. Dry croupy cough which sounds hollow, barking or like a saw. Wakes with a feeling of suffocation. Cough can be brought on by talking or by a dry, cold wind. Difficulty in coughing up phlegm, so swallows it (Causticum). Burning, rawness and weakness in chest. Bitter taste in throat. The person must lie down, they feel exhausted.

Areas of application Asthma. Croup. Whooping cough.

Pain Tightness in chest; violent palpitation with suffocating cough.

Worse Before midnight. Dry, cold wind. Warm room. Lying down with head low (Pulsatilla). If woken up. Full moon.

Better Warm drinks and food.

Staphysagria
Delphinium staphysagria
Stavesacre

This plant is a species of larkspur indigenous to southern Europe and its seeds are extremely poisonous. It has been used to kill parasites, to cause vomiting, and to relieve toothache, itching and warts. In poisonings it has caused paralysis of the spinal cord and death from asphyxia.

Characteristic symptoms The essence of this remedy seems to lie in its sensitivity to invasion of space – of mind, emotions or body: children bullied at school; people under 'attack' in some way (who don't fight back but smoulder away inside, having an occasional outburst of anger). Or an unwanted visitor arrives and is tolerated by much holding of the tongue! Surgery, especially to abdomen, reproductive organs, anus or bladder. Vaginal examinations. Feeling of invasion after sex. 'Honeymoon' cystitis (burning in bladder region when *not* passing urine). Clean-cut wounds and pain which remains after surgery. Anger and feelings of indignation with trembling. Colic after operations or brought on after anger (this can be colic in a breastfed baby whose parents become angry).

Areas of application Abortion. After surgery, medical examinations. Bites. Colic. Cystitis. Headlice. Morning sickness. Resentment and anger, not expressed directly. Shingles. Styes. Tearfulness.

Pain Stinging. Stitching. Smarting. Squeezing. Cramp. Sharp, as if stabbed by knife.

Worse Touch. Emotions. Suppressed anger.

Better Warmth. Rest. Breakfast.

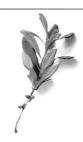
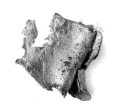
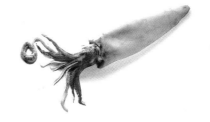

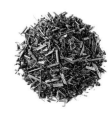

Sulphur

Brimstone, Flowers of sulphur

Sulphur is a product of volcanic eruptions and has been used for at least 2,000 years to treat skin disorders. It occurs in nature as a crystalline solid and is found in all living tissue.

Characteristic symptoms Mentally full of ideas but has difficulty in delivering the end product. Tend to be self-centred, untidy, sluggish people who would prefer to sit rather than stand. They are always too hot and walk around in the winter with minimal clothing on. Hot and sweaty in bed and stick their feet out from under the bedclothes. Huge appetites, suddenly get hungry and weak about 11 a.m.; or instead of eating they have insatiable thirst. Love sweets, dislike meat. Disturbed circulation brings **Brimstone** on burning, flushes of heat, and redness of ears, lips, nose, anus. Nasal catarrh is blocked when indoors. Like to have catnaps.

Areas of application At the end of an acute illness when the person does not fully recover. Bronchitis. Coughs. Colds. Diarrhoea. Earache. Measles. Throat. Vertigo.

Pain Burning. Throbbing. Stitching pain which goes through from chest to back.

Worse Washing and having a bath. At night. From warmth of bed. 11 a.m. Standing. Over-exertion. Milk.

Better Open air. Sitting, leaning.

CAUTION: Use with great care. If there is a history of skin complaints, avoid self-prescribing it, as aggravations can result.

Symphytum

Symphytum officinalis
Boneset, Comfrey, Knitbone

This plant is a native of Europe and Asia, and prefers wet places such as banks of rivers and ditches. Its use in the Middle Ages was widespread for broken bones. The botanical name is from Greek 'symphyo', meaning to unite. The juice of the root is glutinous and, according to Gerarde, 'It will solder and glue together meat that is chopped in pieces, seething in a pot, and make it in one lump.'

Characteristic symptoms Symphytum causes bone to grow and so promotes the fast healing of fractures. Use for injuries to hard parts of the body such as the periostum (bone covering). (Arnica for soft parts.) Painful swellings without discoloration (Arnica for obvious bruising). Pain in eyeball after injuries. Pain in stump after amputation (*see also* Hypericum).

Areas of application Episiotomy. Fractures. Painful stump after amputations. Wounds that don't knit back together.

Pain Pricking, stitching.

Worse Injuries, especially from blunt instruments. Touch.

CAUTION: Do not use this remedy if a pin has been used in a broken bone.

Tabacum

Nicotiana tabacum
Tobacco

The French Ambassador to Portugal, Jean Nicot, gave his name to the tobacco plant, which was taken to France around 1560. Originally from South America, it was brought to Europe by Columbus. It is known to have detrimental effects on the digestion, circulation and heart, causing nausea and vomiting and drowsiness. It has been used as an insecticide and rubbed on bee stings and mosquito bites to bring relief. Vinegar and sour apples antidote the effects of raw tobacco.

Characteristic symptoms Extreme giddiness with profuse cold sweat. Seasickness with sinking feeling in stomach as if they will faint. Nausea which is much worse from the smell of tobacco. Vomits from the smallest movement. Wants abdomen uncovered, which relieves.

Areas of application Bee stings and

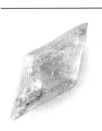
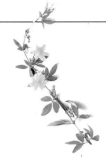

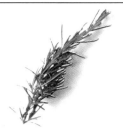

mosquito bites. Nausea and vomiting in pregnancy. Travel sickness.

Pain Cramps.

Worse Slightest movement. Motion of cars, ships. Opening eyes. Extremes of heat and cold.

Better Open air. Vomiting. Uncovering the abdomen. Cold applications. Eating sour apples.

Tarentula
Tarentula cubensis
Cuban tarantula

The name tarantula refers to several poisonous spiders; in homeopathy we use two of them: the Spanish and the Cuban. The Cuban spider is the one used for physical complaints.

Characteristic symptoms Abscesses, boils, carbuncles, swellings of any kind – especially on the back of the neck – where skin turns red/blue or purple, with agonizing pain. Deep septic conditions with hardness of the affected part and sudden loss of vitality, with sweating. (Compare Arsenicum and Carbo Veg.) Symptoms come on suddenly and may return annually. Sleepless, restless with fidgety feet.

Areas of application Abscesses. Carbuncles. Plague. Septic conditions.

Pain Burning. Stinging. Throbbing. Pricking like needles.

Worse Night. Annually. Noise. Touch.

Better Smoking tobacco. Open air.

Urtica Urens
Lesser nettle, Stinging nettle

The lesser nettle has almost identical properties to the common nettle (U. dioica) and the same habitat. It has been used for urinary problems, as a blood cleanser, hair restorative and as an antidote to poisonous plants and insect bites. In homeopathy it was renowned for its use in gout and removing gravel in the urine.

Lesser nettle

Characteristic symptoms Itching, stinging pain and swellings, particularly blistery swellings (compare Apis). For burns apply diluted tincture immediately, as well as taking the remedy in tablet form. It promotes the flow of breast milk and can have the opposite effect when the woman decides to stop breastfeeding. Apply neat to bee stings. Use in cystitis where the urine burns the skin and there is difficulty passing it.

Areas of application Allergies to shellfish. Bee stings. Breast milk lacking, or weaning. Burns. Cystitis.

Pain Stinging. Burning.

Worse Touch.

Veratrum Alb
Veratrum album
White hellebore

Found growing in Europe, this extremely poisonous plant has been used for tipping arrows and daggers. If eaten, it causes severe vomiting and diarrhoea with sweating and fainting, which may continue into convulsions and death. It was used in Greek times for purging the body in spring and autumn, and Hahnemann used it, Cuprum and Camphor with great success in outbreaks of cholera.

Characteristic symptoms Excessive purging – retching, vomiting, diarrhoea and sweating (especially on the forehead). The person is very cold, with a bluish face. Diarrhoea may come on after drinking cold water on a hot day. Violent pains in colic with cramps in the legs; cramps anywhere. Children like to be carried quickly. Crave ice-water which is vomited immediately. (Phosphorus warms up in stomach.) Violent thirst.

Areas of application Colic. Collapse. Diarrhoea. Fainting. Nausea, vomiting.

Pain Cutting. Cramp.

Worse Drinking. Cold drinks. Fruit.

Better Warmth. Hot drinks. Milk.

AILMENT	SYMPTOMS/DETAIL	REMEDY (Internal unless specified)
BITES AND STINGS	Bee, hornet, wasp	*Apis, Arnica, Cantharis, Hypericum, Ledum, Urtica Urens* *External: Calendula, Hypercal or Urtica Urens*
	Dog, cat, horse, rat	*Arnica, Belladonna, Echinacea, Hypericum, Ledum*
	Gnat, horsefly, mosquito	*Apis, Cantharis, Hypericum, Ledum*
	Jellyfish	*Arnica, Hypericum, Ledum, Medusa*
	Scorpion, snake, spider	*Arnica, Carbolic Acid, Crotalus Horridus, Echinacea, Lachesis, Ledum*
BLEEDING	From injury	*Arnica, Hamamelis*
	Small wounds	*External: Calendula, Hypercal or Hamamelis*
	Small wounds that bleed profusely	*Phosphorus*
	After surgery	*Carbo Veg, Phosphorus*
BONES	Broken (use after bone is set)	*Calc Phos, Symphytum*
	Broken ribs	*Bryonia*
	Bruised	*Arnica, Calc Phos, Ruta, Symphytum*
	Bruised bone covering (shin)	*Ruta*
BREATHING DIFFICULTIES	Allergic reaction	*Apis, Carbolic Acid, Crotalus Horridus*
	Asthma	*Arsenicum, Carbo Veg*
	As if drowning in own secretions (mucus)	*Ant Tart*
	Newborn baby	*Ant Tart, Carbo Veg*
BRUISES		*Arnica, Bellis Perennis*
	Breast	*Bellis Perennis*
	Eyeball	*Symphytum*
	Nerve-rich parts	*Bellis Perennis, Hypericum*
BURNS	Minor	*Urtica Urens (and externally)*
	Serious	*Cantharis, Carbo Veg, Causticum*
	Suppurating	*Calc Sulph*
COLLAPSE	Sudden	*Arsenicum, Phosphorus*
	After diarrhoea	*Arsenicum, Carbo Veg, Veratrum Alb*
	Bite of poisonous insects and animals	*Apis, Carbolic Acid, Crotalus Horridus*
CUTS AND WOUNDS	Crushed fingers and toes	*Hypericum*
	Inflamed	*Hepar Sulph, Silica*
	Festering with pus	*Hepar Sulph, Silica*
	Continuous oozing of pus	*Calc Sulph*
	Lacerated	*Calendula, Hamamelis, Hypericum, Staphysagria*
	Punctured (rusty nail, barbed wire)	*Arnica, Hypericum, Ledum*
	Unhealthy, won't heal	*Calc Sulph, Silica*
EYES	Black eye	*Arnica*
	Eyeball	*Symphytum*

AILMENT	SYMPTOMS/DETAIL	REMEDY (Internal unless specified)
EYES (cont.)	After foreign object removed	*Hypericum*
	Bleeding	*Externally: Calendula*
FAINTING	From blood loss	*China*
	From excitement	*Coffea*
	From hot room	*Pulsatilla*
	From lights	*Nux Vomica*
	From pain	*Apis, Chamomilla, Hepar Sulph, Nux Vomica*
FROSTBITE	Blue skin, worse heat	*Lachesis*
	Needle-like pain	*Agaricus*
	Stinging pain, worse heat	*Apis*
HEAD	Injury	*Arnica*
	Headache after injury	*Nat Sulph*
NOSEBLEED		*Arnica, Carbo Veg, Hamamelis, Ipecac, Lachesis, Phosphorus*
	Bright red	*Ipecac, Phosphorus*
	Dark blood	*Carbo Veg, Hamamelis, Lachesis*
	Gushing	*Ipecac*
	Instead of monthly period	*Phosphorus*
PAIN	Intolerable ('can't bear it')	*Chamomilla*
	Fear of touch	*Arnica*
	Bruised, sore	*Arnica, Bellis Perennis, Hamamelis, Ruta*
	Shooting	*Belladonna, Hypericum*
	Throbbing	*Belladonna*
	(see also Cramp, page 88)	
SHOCK	With fear, restlessness	*Aconite*
	Any shock	*Arnica*
SPRAINS AND STRAINS	Muscles	*Arnica, Rhus Tox*
	Joints	*Arnica, Bryonia, Ledum, Rhus Tox*
	Tendons, ligaments	*Rhus Tox, Ruta*
SUNBURN	see Burns	
SUNSTROKE	Shock and fear	*Aconite*
	Throbbing headache:	*Belladonna, Glonoine*
	better bending head back	*Belladonna*
	worse bending head back	*Glonione*
TETANUS	Preventative	*Hypericum, Ledum*

AILMENT	SYMPTOMS/DETAIL	REMEDY (Internal unless specified)
BRONCHITIS	Early stages	*Aconite, Ferrum Phos*
	After exposure to cold, dry wind	*Aconite, Hepar Sulph*
	Burning, tight chest; worse talking, laughing	*Phosphorus*
	Dry, painful cough, stitching pain, worse moving	*Bryonia*
	Loose, rattling cough	*Ant Tart, Hepar Sulph*
	Chest full of phlegm: worse warm drinks worse cold drinks	*Ant Tart* *Hepar Sulph*
	Worse in heated room	*Pulsatilla*
CHICKEN POX	Early stages with fever and restlessness	*Aconite*
	Rash develops slowly with rattly chest	*Ant Tart*
	Very high fever with flushed face	*Belladonna*
	Weepy child, worse alone; thirstless	*Pulsatilla*
	Worse at night, very itchy, restless, chilly	*Rhus Tox*
COLDS	Sudden onset after exposure to cold winds	*Aconite*
	Burning, watery cold; can't get warm	*Arsenicum*
	Sneezing first, goes to chest; with burning headache; better in moist, cool air	*Bryonia*
	Summer colds, or gets wet and cold on a hot day	*Dulcamara*
COUGHS	Worse from cold, dry winds	*Aconite*
	Burning chest; feels better outdoors	*Sulphur*
	Dry, barking with headache	*Bryonia*
	Weakness prevents raising phlegm	*Causticum*
CROUP	After exposure to cold, dry winds; barking cough; restless, anxious	*Aconite*
	Whistling breathing; gasps for breath; better warm drinks	*Spongia*
	Loose, rattly cough; worse uncovering	*Hepar Sulph*
CYSTITIS	Burning, stinging pain; thirstless	*Apis*
	Stabbing pain, worse before and after urinating	*Cantharis*
	Painful retention after surgery, or cold weather	*Causticum*
	Ineffectual urging	*Nux Vomica*
	After operations to sexual organs, or sexual activity	*Staphysagria*
EARACHE	Sudden, from cold, dry wind	*Aconite*
	Screams with pain; external ear red	*Apis*
	Throbbing pain with high fever	*Belladonna*
	With teething in bad-tempered child	*Chamomilla*
	Pain moves from throat to ear on swallowing	*Hepar Sulph*
	During air travel	*Kali Mur*
	With discharge; tearful, clingy child; worse warmth	*Pulsatilla*
	Sensitive to cold; perforated eardrum	*Silica*

ACUTE ILLNESS (cont.)		
AILMENT	**SYMPTOMS/DETAIL**	**REMEDY** (Internal unless specified)
FEVER	Early onset after cold, dry winds	*Aconite*
	Anxious, weak, restless	*Arsenicum*
	Delirious; flushed face; dry, burning skin	*Belladonna*
	Early stages; throbbing	*Ferrum Phos*
	Thirstless, tearful children who like cuddles	*Pulsatilla*
	Thirst for very cold drinks; hunger with fever	*Phosphorus*
FLU		*Arsenicum, Baptisia, Bryonia, Dulcamara, Eupatorium Perf, Gelsemium, Nux Vomica, Rhus Tox*
	Aching bones as if broken	*Eupatorium Perf*
	Aching muscles	*Gelsemium*
	Aching eyeballs	*Bryonia, Eupatorium Perf, Gelsemium*
MEASLES	At beginning with fever and restlessness	*Aconite*
	Bright red rash; dry, burning heat	*Belladonna*

	Catarrhal symptoms:
	   streaming, burning tears; bland nasal discharge
	   thick yellow bland discharge from eyes which itch and burn
		Euphrasia
		Pulsatilla

	Heavy head, drowsy, thirstless	*Gelsemium*
MUMPS	Right-sided; violent pain; high fever	*Belladonna*
	Left-sided; worse at night	*Rhus Tox*
	Offensive sweat and breath	*Merc Sol*
	Pain shoots to ear on swallowing	*Phytolacca*
	Moves to breasts, ovaries, testicles	*Carbo Veg, Pulsatilla*
SEPTIC CONDITIONS	Heavy, sore, aching muscles; confused, restless	*Baptisia*
	Aching, weak, slow – after bites, stings	*Echinacea*
	Chronic complaints from septic states	*Pyrogen*
TEETHING	Vomits milk immediately after feeding	*Aethusa*
	Hot flushed face, light sensitive	*Belladonna*
	Unbearable pain; nothing pleases	*Chamomilla*
	Worse at night; much dribbling	*Merc Sol*
THROAT	After being in cold, dry wind	*Aconite*
	Drowsy, as if drugged; dark red throat; heavy, aching muscles	*Baptisia*
	Burning throat; better warm drinks	*Arsenicum*
	Burning, stinging pain; better cold drinks	*Apis*
	From damp, cold weather; colds settle in throat	*Dulcamara*
	Inflamed, bright red throat; 'strawberry' tongue; congested; hot, red face	*Belladonna*
WHOOPING COUGH	Cries before cough	*Arnica*
	Bright red in face on coughing	*Belladonna*
	Suffocating cough, with nosebleed	*Ipecac*

NON-ACUTE FIRST AID

AILMENT	SYMPTOMS/DETAIL	REMEDY (Internal unless specified)
ABSCESSES, BOILS, CARBUNCLES	Stinging, burning pain, worse heat	*Apis*
	Crops of boils do not mature	*Arnica*
	Burning, stabbing pain, better warmth	*Arsenicum*
	Threatening abscess with throbbing pain	*Belladonna*
	Much thick yellow pus	*Calc Sulph*
	Sharp, splinter-like pain	*Hepar Sulph*
	Slow development; may result in hard lumps	*Silica*
CHILBLAINS	Hot or cold needle pain	*Agaricus*
	Redness, heat and swelling	*Ferrum Phos*
	Itches more in warm room	*Pulsatilla*
COLD SORES	Burning, stinging pain	*Arsenicum*
	With pus; worse for touch	*Hepar Sulph*
	Watery blisters on lips	*Nat Mur*
CRAMP		*Chamomilla, Colocynth, Cuprum, Lycopodium, Mag Phos, Nux Vomica, Sulphur*
	Calf muscles; while in bed	*Causticum, Hepar Sulph, Nux Vomica, Rhus Tox, Sepia, Sulphur*
	While sitting	*Rhus Tox*
	In fingers while writing; playing musical instrument	*Mag Phos*
EYESTRAIN	Red, burning, sore, watery eyes	*Euphrasia (and externally)*
	Hot, red, painful from overuse, e.g. computer work; dim vision	*Ruta*
HAYFEVER	Burning nasal discharge; bland eye secretions	*Allium Cepa*
	Red, burning, itchy, sore eyes	*Euphrasia (and externally)*
HEADACHES	From injury	*Arnica, Nat Sulph*
	At weekends, or from excitement	*Arsenicum*
	Sudden throbbing pain, with light sensitivity	*Belladonna*
MOUTH ULCERS (CANKER SORES)	White ulcers, white tongue	*Kali Mur*
	With offensive breath	*Merc Sol*
	Blisters and ulcers in mouth and on tongue	*Nat Mur*
PILES	Rectum feels full of sticks; sharp shooting pain	*Aesculus*
	After childbirth	*Arnica*
	Splinter, needle pain	*Nit Ac*
	Burning, itching, worse warmth of bed, or from standing	*Sulphur*
STYES	Stinging pain, worse heat	*Apis*
	Splinter pain, worse cold	*Hepar Sulph*
	Slow to ripen	*Silica*
	Recurrent, especially where anger is unexpressed	*Staphysagria*

DENTIST & SURGERY

AILMENT	SYMPTOMS/DETAIL	REMEDY (Internal unless specified)
ANAESTHETICS	Drowsy after	Gelsemium, Phosphorus
	Mental confusion	Gelsemium
	As a preventative for nausea and vomiting after general anaesthetic	Phosphorus
	Morphine, pethidine	Chamomilla, Coffea, Nux Vomica
	Ergometrine, syntometrine (childbirth)	Secale
FEAR AND PANIC		see Pregnancy & Childbirth table, page 91
HAEMORRHAGE	As a preventative before any operation	Arnica
	After tooth extraction	Hamamelis Externally: Calendula or Hypercal
	Heavy bleeding from small wounds	Phosphorus
	From injury	Arnica
	Sudden collapse	Carbo Veg
	With nausea	Ipecac
PAIN		see Accidents and Emergencies table, page 85; Cramp, page 88
TOOTH ABSCESS	Burning pain, better heat	Arsenicum
	Much yellow pus	Calc Sulph
	Stinging pain, worse heat	Apis
	Sharp, stabbing pain	Hepar Sulph
	Brings pus to the surface	Silica
	Violent throbbing	Belladonna

TRAVEL

AILMENT	SYMPTOMS/DETAIL	REMEDY (Internal unless specified)
JETLAG		Arnica, Belladona
JET TRAVEL	Ear pain	Kali Mur, Silica
	Swollen feet and ankles	Nat Mur, Nat Phos, Nat Sulph
FEAR		Aconite, Arg Nit, Gelsemium
IMPURE WATER		China, Echinacea – dissolve tablets in or add a few drops of tincture to drinking water
SICKNESS	Better indoors, lying down	Cocculus
	Better head high; worse open air	Petroleum
	Better fresh air; worse opening eyes	Tabacum

DIGESTIVE DISTURBANCES

AILMENT	SYMPTOMS/DETAIL	REMEDY (Internal unless specified)
COLIC	Breast-fed babies, from mother eating spicy food	*Nux Vomica*
	From anger	*Chamomilla, Colocynth, Staphysagria*
	Worse eating sweets	*Sulphur*
	Worse after being punished or bullied	*Staphysagria*
	Better bending double	*Colocynth*
	Better stretching out or bending backwards	*Dioscorea*
CONSTIPATION	With bursting headache	*Bryonia*
	Light-coloured stools	*Kali Mur*
	When away from home	*Lycopodium*
	Dry, hard stools; craves salt	*Nat Mur*
	Desire to empty bowels but can't	*Nux Vomica*
DIARRHOEA	After the following:	
	Beer	*Lycopodium, Sulphur*
	Breakfast	*Arg Nit, Lycopodium, Nux Vomica, Phosphorus*
	Coffee	*Phosphorus*
	Drugs	*Nux Vomica*
	Excitement	*Arg Nit, Gelsemium, Lycopodium*
	Fatty food	*Carbo Veg, Pulsatilla*
	Fright	*Aconite, Arg Nit, Gelsemium, Phosphorus, Pulsatilla*
	Fruit	*Arsenicum, China, Colocynth, Lycopodium, Nat Sulph, Pulsatilla*
	Milk	*Lycopodium, Sepia, Sulphur*
	Pork	*Pulsatilla*
	Shellfish	*Carbo Veg*
	Sugar	*Arg Nit*
	In morning, driving from bed	*Sulphur*
	During teething	*Aconite, Chamomilla, Merc Sol, Sulphur*
FLATULENCE	Post-operative	*Carbo Veg, China*
	After rich, fatty food	*Carbo Veg*
	Constant belching, no relief	*China*
	Constant belching gives relief	*Carbo Veg*
	Loud rumbling from onions, beans	*Lycopodium*
INDIGESTION	After alcohol	*Nux Vomica*
	After rich, fatty food	*Carbo Veg, Nux Vomica, Pulsatilla*
	Heaviness in stomach, abdomen	*Sulphur*
	Weight like a stone in stomach	*Pulsatilla*
HEARTBURN		*Lycopodium, Nat Mur, Nat Phos, Nat Sulph*
	Burning rises to throat	*Lycopodium*
	Burning eructations	*Nat Mur*
	Sour eructations	*Nat Phos*
NAUSEA	Continuous	*Ipecac, Nux Vomica, Phosphorus, Silica*
	No relief from vomiting	*Ipecac*
	Desire to vomit but can't; clean tongue	*Nux Vomica*
	From warm drinks	*Phosphorus, Pulsatilla*

DIGESTIVE DISTURBANCES (cont.)

AILMENT	SYMPTOMS/DETAIL	REMEDY (Internal unless specified)
NAUSEA (cont.)	From cold drinks	Arsenicum, Cuprum, Lycopodium, Nat Mur, Nux Vomica, Pulsatilla
	From smell of food	Arsenicum, Ipecac, Sepia
	From rich food	Ipecac, Pulsatilla, Sepia
	Before breakfast	Sepia, Lycopodium
VOMITING	Food poisoning	Arsenicum
	When food and drink warm up in stomach	Phosphorus
	Of food eaten much earlier	Pulsatilla
	Excessive purging from stomach and bowels with cold sweat on forehead	Veratrum Alb
	Violent vomiting in pregnancy with diarrhoea	Aethusa, Arsenicum, Veratrum Alb
	After anger	Chamomilla, Colocynth, Nux Vomica

PRENANCY & CHILDBIRTH

AILMENT	SYMPTOMS/DETAIL	REMEDY (Internal unless specified)
AFTER-PAINS	In groin	Cimicifuga
	Very tearful, better for company	Pulsatilla
	Restless, better moving	Rhus Tox
	Severe, in sacrum and hips after forceps delivery	Hypericum
BABY'S MOVEMENTS	Nausea and vomiting from movements	Arnica
	Unbearable	Arnica, Sepia
BACKACHE	After forceps delivery	Rhus Tox
	After strain of childbirth	Rhus Tox
	During and after posterior labour	Kali Carb
	During pregnancy with dragging down feeling	Sepia
BREASTFEEDING	To dry milk up	Lac Can, Pulsatilla, Urtica Urens
	To increase milk supply	Lac Can, Pulsatilla, Urtica Urens
	Pain during	Silica
	Tearful during	Pulsatilla
	Nipples cracked	Castor Equi, Hepar Sulph
	Mastitis	Belladonna, Bryonia, Phytolacca
CAESAREAN		see Dentist & Surgery table, page 89; Pain, page 85
	Before and after operation	Arnica

AILMENT	SYMPTOMS/DETAIL	REMEDY (Internal unless specified)
CAESAREAN (cont.)	Before general anaesthetic (to prevent nausea and vomiting)	Phosphorus
EPIDURAL	Pain along nerve pathways	Hypericum
EPISIOTOMY	Burning, raw, sore pain	Causticum
	Burning, sharp, cutting pain	Staphysagria
FAINTING	In a warm room	Pulsatilla
	From bright lights	Nux Vomica
	From labour pains	Nux Vomica
FEAR	Nervous excitement	Gelsemium
	Being alone	Phosphorus, Pulsatilla
	Suddenly going into labour	Aconite, Arnica
	Of dying	Aconite, Arsenicum
FORCEPS	Violent pains in sacrum	Hypericum
	Feels violated	Staphysagria
HAEMORRHAGE	From injury	Arnica
	Profuse bleeding from small area	Phosphorus
LABOUR	Rapid onset; shock; bruising	Arnica
	Exhaustion from prolonged labour	Caulophyllum
	Slow progress	Caulophyllum
	Intolerable pain ('can't bear it')	Chamomilla
	Wants to give up ('can't do it')	Cimicifuga
	Heaviness with pains extending to the back	Gelsemium
	Prefers to be alone	Nat Mur
	Prefers company	Phosphorus, Pulsatilla
	Irritable, fault-finding, feels cold	Nux Vomica
	Talks through contractions	Cimicifuga
PROLAPSE	Womb, after forceps	Secale
	Rectum, after birth	Ruta
VARICOSE VEINS	During or after pregnancy	Bellis Perennis, Pulsatilla, Hamamelis
WALKING DIFFICULTIES	During pregnancy	Bellis Perennis

Remedy Names & Abbreviations

ABBREVIATED NAME	FULL NAME	COMMON NAME
Aconite, Acon	Aconitum Napellus	Monkshood, Wolfsbane
Aesculus, Aesc	Aesculus Hippocastanum	Horse chestnut tree
Aethusa, Aeth	Aethusa Cynapium	Fool's parsley
Agaricus, Agar	Agaricus Muscarius	Fly agaric, Toadstool
Al Cepa	Allium Cepa	Common red onion
Anacardium, Anac	Anacardium Orientale	Malacca nut, Marking nut
Ant Crud	Antimonium Crudum	Sulphide of antimony
Ant Tart	Antimonium Tartaricum	Tartar emetic
Apis	Apis Mellifica	Honey bee
Arg Nit	Argenticum Nitricum	Nitrate of silver
Arnica, Arn	Arnica Montana	Leopard's bane, Mountain tobacco
Arsenicum, Arsen Alb	Arsenicum Album	White oxide of metallic arsenic
Baptisia, Bapt	Baptisia Tinctoria	Wild indigo
Belladonna, Bell	Atropa Belladonna	Deadly nightshade
Bellis Perennis		Common daisy
Bryonia	Bryonia Alba	Wild hops
Calc Carb	Calcarea Carbonica	Calcium carbonate, carbonate of lime
Calc Fluor	Calcarea Fluorica	Fluoride of lime, Fluorspar
Calc Phos	Calcarea Phosphorica	Phosphate of lime
Calc Sulph	Calcarea Sulphurica	Gypsum, Plaster of Paris
Calendula	Calendula Officinalis	Marigold
Cantharis	Cantharis Vesicatoria	Spanish fly
Carbo Veg	Carbo Vegetabilis	Wood charcoal
Carbolic Acid	Carbolicum Acidum	Carbolic acid
Castor Equi		Horse's thumbnail
Caulophyllum	Caulophyllum Thalictroides	Blue cohosh, Squaw root
Causticum		Potassium hydrate
Chamomilla	Matricaria Chamomilla	German chamomile
China	China Officinalis	Cinchona bark Peruvian bark
Cimicifuga	Actea Racemosa	Black cohosh
Cocculus	Cocculus Indicus	Fish berry, India berry
Coccus Cacti		Cochineal
Coffea	Coffea Cruda	Coffee, Mocha bean
Colocynth	Colocynthis	Bitter apple, Bitter cucumber
Crotalus Horridus		Rattlesnake
Cuprum	Cuprum Metallicum	Copper
Drosera	Drosera Rotundifolia	Sundew
Dulcamara	Solanum Dulcamara	Bittersweet, Woody nightshade
Echinacea	Echinacea Angustifolia	Purple cone flower
Eupatorium Perf	Eupatorium Perfoliatum	Boneset, Indian sage
Euphrasia	Euphrasia Officinalis	Eyebright

ABBREVIATED NAME	FULL NAME	COMMON NAME
Ferrum Phos	Ferrum Phosphoricum	White phosphate of iron
Gelsemium	Gelsemium Sempervirens	Yellow jasmine
Glonoine		Nitroglycerine
Hamamelis	Hamamelis Virginica	Witch hazel
Hepar Sulph	Hepar Sulphuris Calcareum	Sulphide of calcium
Hypericum	Hypericum Perfoliatum	St John's wort
Ignatia	Ignatia Amara	St Ignatia's bean
Ipecac	Cephaelis Ipecacuanha	Ipecacuanha
Kali Bic	Kali Bichromicum	Bichromate of potash
Kali Carb	Kali Carbonicum	Potassium carbonate
Kali Mur	Kali Muriaticum	Potassium chloride
Kali Phos	Kali Phosphoricum	Potassium phosphate
Kali Sulph	Kali Sulphuricum	Potassium sulphate
Lachesis	Trigonocephalus Lachesis	Bushmaster, surukuku snake
Ledum	Ledum Palustre	Wild rosemary
Lycopodium	Lycopodium Clavatum	Clubmoss, Wolf's claw
Mag Phos	Magnesium Phosphoricum	Magnesium phosphate
Merc Sol	Mercurius Solubilis	Mercury, quicksilver
Mezereum	Daphne Mezereum	Spurge olive
Nat Mur	Natrum Muriaticum	Sodium chloride, common salt
Nat Phos	Natrum Phosphoricum	Sodium phosphate
Nat Sulph	Natrum Sulphuricum	Sodium sulphate
Nit Ac	Nitricum Acidum	Nitric acid
Nux Vomica	Strychnos Nux Vomica	Poison nut
Petroleum	Oleum Petrae	Crude rock oil
Phosphorus		the element
Phytolacca	Phytolacca Decandra	Poke root
Pulsatilla	Pulsatilla Nigricans	Meadow anemone, Pasque flower, wind flower
Pyrogen	Pyrogenium	Sepsin
Rhus Tox	Rhus Toxicondendron	Poison ivy
Ruta	Ruta Graveolens	Rue
Secale	Secale Cornutum	Ergot of rye
Sepia	Sepia Officinalis	Cuttlefish, squid
Silica	Silica Terra	Flint
Spongia	Spongia Tosta	Roasted sea sponge
Staphysagria	Delphinium taphysagria	Stavesacre
Sulphur		Brimstone, flowers of sulphur
Symphytum	Symphytum Officinalis	Boneset, comfrey, knitbone
Tabacum	Nicotiana Tabacum	Tobacco
Tarentula	Tarentula Cubensis	Cuban tarantula
Urtica Urens		Lesser nettle, stinging nettle
Veratrum Alb	Veratrum Album	White hellebore

Glossary

Abortion This word has come to mean a deliberately induced termination of pregnancy.

Acute illness Normally a short-lasting illness with a rapid onset. Recovery often takes place with no medical intervention.

Allopathy Orthodox medicine, which uses substances to produce opposite effects, such as prescribing laxatives to help constipation.

Antidote Anything which reduces or spoils the effect of a homeopathic remedy.

Atony Lack of tone in a particular organ or muscle.

Bach Flower Remedies These are prepared from a variety of plants, including bushes and trees. The system of 38 remedies was formulated in the 1930s by Dr Edward Bach, a homeopath and bacteriologist.

Chronic illness Long-lasting disorders which come on gradually and lead to a weakened state of health. They may follow on from an acute illness where the person has not fully recovered. Healing intervention is normally necessary.

Congenital A condition which is present from birth. It can be inherited, or result from injury sustained in the womb.

Constitutional prescribing This procedure is undertaken during a consultation with a professional homeopath in which remedies are chosen to match a fully documented personal history.

Dentition The cutting of teeth.

Engorgement Congested, filled to excess.

Episiotomy The cutting of the perineum (c.f.) during labour.

Ergometrine A drug given to cause contractions of the uterine muscle during labour.

Eructations Belching

Eruptions An outbreak of a rash on the skin surface.

Fontanelles Soft spots on the top of a baby's head where bone has not yet formed. These normally close by the age of 18 months.

Immune system The body's natural defence mechanism which maintains health. It can be seriously undermined by stress, environmental pollutants, hereditary factors, powerful drugs, immunization, and some habitual thought patterns.

Lassitude Weariness, sleepiness.

Leucorrhoea Literally 'white discharge', but in homeopathy it is taken to describe any vaginal discharge, whether infected or not.

Lochia Normal discharge from the uterus after childbirth.

Maintaining cause A wide range of maintaing causes underlie many complaints, including long-standing sadness, anger, resentment, poor diet, lack of exercise, smoking or excess alcohol (see Immune system above).

Miscarriage This term is commonly used to describe a spontaneous or accidental ending of a pregnancy.

Mother tincture A solution of the active principles of a substance in alcohol, the word 'mother' being used by homeopathic pharmacies. Making a mother tincture is the first stage of making a homeopathic remedy (see page 14).

Mucous membrane A delicate skin-like layer containing glands that secrete mucus (c.f.), e.g. the lining of the nose.

Mucus The slimy secretion derived from mucous membranes (c.f.).

Neuralgia Pain originating in a nerve.

Oedematous A puffy swelling arising from a collection of water.

Ossification The formation of bone. In old age, cartilage may become bone-hard and create brittleness.

Perineum The area of skin and muscle between the genital organs and the anus.

Periosteum Fibrous coating of a bone which is essential for the bone's nutrition.

Phlebitis Inflammation of a vein, which is linked to a blockage caused by a blood clot.

Potency The strength of a remedy, which is determined by the number of terms it has been diluted and succussed (c. f.).

Prolapse Displacement of an organ, such as the rectum or womb, usually from a weakness of the supporting muscles.

Proving The method used in homeopathy for collecting data during the testing of substances on healthy volunteers.

Purulent Containing pus.

Remedies Homeopathic medicines.

Sciatica Pain originating in the sciatic nerve, which runs from the pelvis down the back of the thigh to the calf and foot.

Similimum The homeopathic remedy which most closely resembles a person's symptoms.

Sputum Phlegm or mucus, possibly containing pus, which is coughed up from the air passages.

Succussion The dynamic shaking of remedies during the manufacturing process.

Suppurating Producing pus.

Syntometrine Given routinely by midwives during labour immediately before the baby is delivered, as a means of contracting the uterus to bring about a speedy (unnatural) delivery of the placenta.

Tincture *See* Mother tincture.

Trigeminal neufalgia Severe pain originating in the trigeminal nerve, on the left or right side of the face.

Urticaria Nettle-rash.

Vertigo Giddiness from a disorder of the system.

Vesicles Blisters.

Vulva A woman's external genitals.

Further Reading

The following books are useful to read if you would like to discover more about homeopathy, and alternative health in general.

Arms, Suzanne: *Immaculate Deception*, Bantam Books, 1981.

Blackie, Margery: *The Patient Not the Cure*, Macdonald & Jane's, 1976.

Castro, Miranda: *Homeopathy for Mother and Baby*, Macmillan, 1992.

Chaitow, Leon: *Vaccination and Immunisation: Dangers, Delusions & Alternatives*, C. W. Daniel, 1987.

Coulter, Harris L.: *Homeopathic Science and Modern Medicine: The Physics of Healing With Microdoses*, North Atlantic Books, 1987.

Curtis, Susan: *A Handbook of Homeopathic Alternatives to Immunisation*, Winter Press, 1994.

Hay, Louise: *You Can Heal Your Life*, Eden Grove Editions, 1988.

Harrison, John: *Love Your Disease, It's Keeping You Healthy*, Angus & Robertson Publishers, 1986.

Leboyer, Frederick: *Birth Without Violence*, Fontana, 1977.

Miles, Martin: *Homeopathy and Human Evolution*, Winter Press, 1992.

Moskowitz, Richard: *Homeopathic Medicines for Pregnancy & Childbirth*, North Atlantic Books, 1992.

Neustaeder, Randall: *The Immunisation Decision: A Guide for Parents*, North Atlantic Books, 1992.

Shepherd, Dorothy: *Homeopathy for the First-Aider*, Health Science Press, 1980.

Shepherd, Dorothy: *Homeopathy in Epidemic Diseases*, Health Science Press, 1967.

Shepherd, Dorothy: *The Magic of the Minimum Dose*, Health Science Press, 1964.

Shepherd, Dorothy: *More Magic of the Minimum Dose*, Health Science Press, 1974.

Vithoulkas, George: *Homeopathy, Medicine of the New Man*, Arco Publishing Inc., 1979.

Vithoulkas, George: *The Science of Homeopathy*, Grove Press Inc. 1980

Index